HELPING SOLVE THE U.S. HEALTHCARE CRISIS

The Provider's Guide to Building a Successful Health Plan

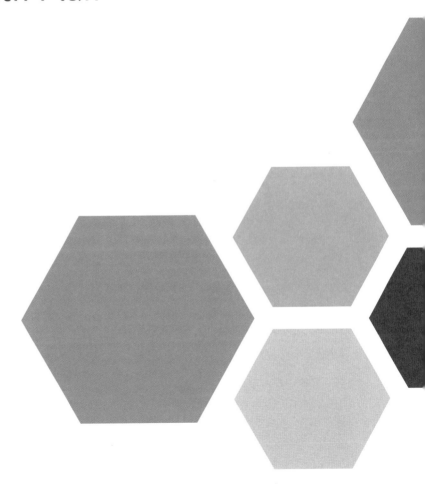

ISBN 978-0-9965856-0-6

HELPING SOLVE THE U.S. HEALTHCARE CRISIS

The Provider's Guide to Building a Successful Health Plan

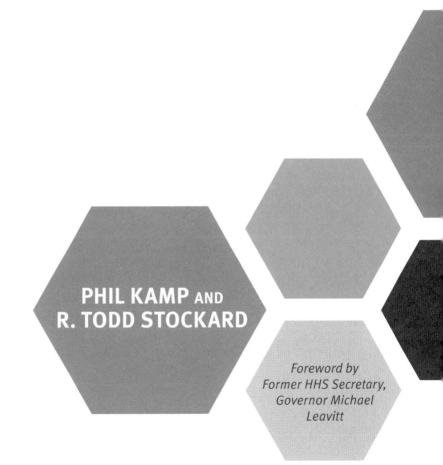

PHIL KAMP AND
R. TODD STOCKARD

*Foreword by
Former HHS Secretary,
Governor Michael
Leavitt*

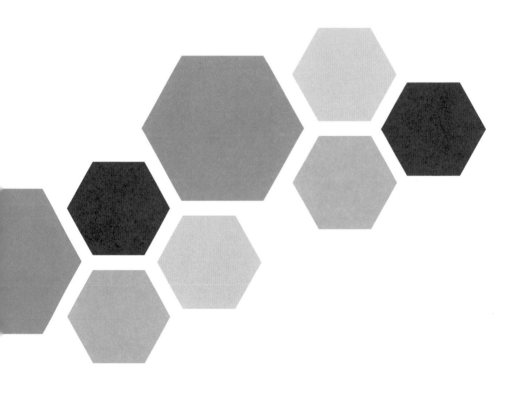

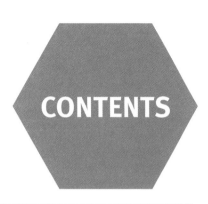

CONTENTS

Acknowledgements

Valence Health always has believed that value-based care is a team sport. That same sentiment also is true when you write a book.

The idea for "Helping Solve the U.S. Healthcare Crisis: The Provider's Guide to Building a Successful Health Plan," literally began in 1996 when the firm (then comprised of five people) worked with George Lynn, President emeritus of AtlanticCare in New Jersey, to help that provider-sponsored health plan (PSHP) get off the ground. After our work with that very first PSHP, we said, "We really should write a book." Following years of experience in the space and much thoughtful consideration, we did just that.

We feel extremely privileged and humbled to have worked alongside so many wonderful healthcare leaders who we also get to call our clients and friends. Their willingness to take leaps of faith and invest in the most complex of all endeavors — the PSHP — continues to inspire us every day.

While we cannot say thank you enough times, we wanted to dedicate a page in the book to acknowledge our clients, staff and friends for getting us where we are and for making the book a reality. Thanks for being part of the Valence Health team!

Enrique Bakemeyer	Mike Coffman	Suzanne Engels
Kylie Barrie	Joe Cecil	Al Ertel
Geri Batten	Lauren Cerra	Lori Fox Ward
Dan Blake	Zachary Cherny	Heidi Furness
Lisa Boero	Steve Cherok	Brett Graham
Nicole Bradberry	Michelle Dary	Devin Gross
Rachel Brand	Shannon Diederich	Lloyd Guthrie
Cheryl Brill	Lou DiGiovine	Anthony Gutierrez
Jason Brown	Ken Dixon	Brandis Hill
Julie Brussow	William Donahue	Allison Hoffman

Stephanie Holland

Shannon McIntyre Hooper

Janet Hughes

Karen Janousek

Jenna King

Angie Kissinger

Daniel Knies

Governor Michael Leavitt

Matthew Levin

Kevin Lewis

Heather Luckenbach

George Lynn

Jessica Martin

Skye McIntyre

J.C. McWilliams

Ashley Merchant

Mark Mixer

Jason Montrie

Jeff Myers

David Nash

Sy Neilson

Kevin Nelson

Deanna Nole

Stephen Nolte

George Pace

Stacey Pearson

Mary Dale Peterson

Sue Price

Julie Randle

Mike Richlen

John Romano

Staci Root

Christopher Roubique

Christine Senty

Robert Sheehy

David Smith

Luke Smith

Ryan Smith

Lon Sprecher

Susan Stein

Lakshmi Subramanian

Gino Tenace

Sara Teppema

Colin Thompson

Tiffany Towery

Steve Tutewohl

Gentre Vartan

Alex Vealitzek

William Wachs

Kevin Weinstein

Shirley Weis

Daniel Yunker

Bill Zimmerman

Foreword

During the aftermath of Hurricane Katrina, I served as U.S. Secretary of Health and Human Services (HHS). The storm destroyed an entire region of the United States. A once vibrant and productive economy virtually ceased to exist, leaving only fragments of a once-thriving and robust business community. Healthcare was no exception, as the natural devastation damaged hospitals, afflicted balance sheets and generated unprecedented healthcare utilization on what remained of the delivery system.

Though the storm brought tragedy and hardship, it also created an opportunity. Within days of the storm, as HHS Secretary, I convened local leaders to begin the process of re-establishing their health system. This was an opportunity to build a more efficient system than what had been in place before the hurricane. The best opportunities for change come in the midst of disruption.

Health reform is disruptive. We are on the front-end of such profound changes in the way the healthcare market works. As such, this is a moment of profound opportunity for improvement.

Employers are re-assessing their long-held social contracts and evaluating new plan options and medical management models. New distribution channels in the form of exchanges are promoting consumerism at a remarkable pace. Unique plan designs, financing mechanisms and network configurations are driving purchasers to change their behavior. Technology companies are transforming the patient-doctor relationship, bearing new forms of clinical utility that are improving health outcomes at lower relative cost. These market forces are driving intense changes for both payors and providers.

The core value proposition for health insurers and other payors is shifting. Traditionally, payors had a comparative advantage by being superior at effectively managing the unpredictability of the underwriting cycle, aggregating lives, administering and supporting members enrolled in plans and managing risk through data and management protocols. Each of these hallmark functions are under some type of pressure. Underwriting fell victim to the Affordable Care Act. Distribution and enrollment can now be conducted through exchanges. Third-party entities and Software-as-a-Service solutions abound to lower relative administrative costs. Risk management responsibilities are slowly being diffused throughout the system, with providers bearing a wider range of risk profiles.

On our current path, I suspect we will see two types of payors in the future: payors who are operated as regulated utilities, and payors who either own care assets or are an asset to a provider organization.

Care providers are undergoing a period of rapid change as a combination of policy and market-driven incentives, programs and activities are converging to establish provider-sponsored "value" in the marketplace. If the expectation set of purchasers is indeed changing, the market will place a premium on such provider enhancements. Thus, the providers' push to invest in new operating models will allow them to bear and manage the risk associated with caring for a patient population.

The end-point for such transformation will vary and be contingent on market dynamics, institutional ethos, community sentiments and an underlying economic shift. From shared savings, to bundles and capitated arrangements, there are several reimbursement schemes to adopt that promote this change. The pinnacle of provider risk-bearing, however, is the full-on establishment of a health plan.

This is not a small undertaking and should be treated with the gravity it deserves. That said, the capacity to establish the traditional functions of payors is becoming within reach for organizations with sufficient capital and a capacity to influence the way care is provided.

The new solutions in distribution, administration and risk management can change the proposition for the right providers to establish a plan that provides unique competitive advantages while concurrently driving systemic value.

In the pages that follow, Valence Health lays out thoughtful considerations in evaluating a more rapid evolution along the risk spectrum. For those who decide to pursue a provider-sponsored health plan, this book outlines strategies, tools and other considerations.

Every healthcare stakeholder should take a deeply strategic look at its market and inventory methods to create greater value. The creation of that value will move market share, bend cost curves and ultimately establish a uniquely American health system; one we should all aspire to.

Michael O. Leavitt

Michael O. Leavitt
Leavitt Partners, Chairman

U.S. Secretary of Health and Human Services (2005–2009)
Administrator, U.S. Environmental Protection Agency (2003–2005)
Governor, State of Utah (1993–2003)

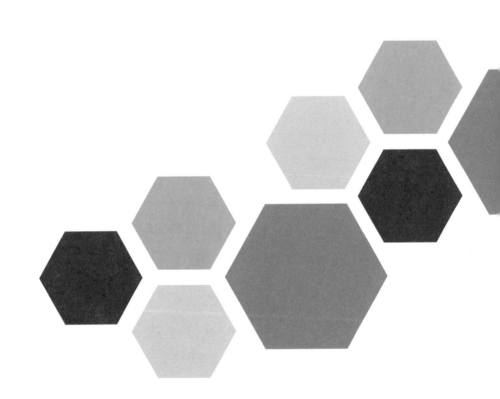

Part One

WHY BECOME A PROVIDER-SPONSORED HEALTH PLAN (PSHP)?

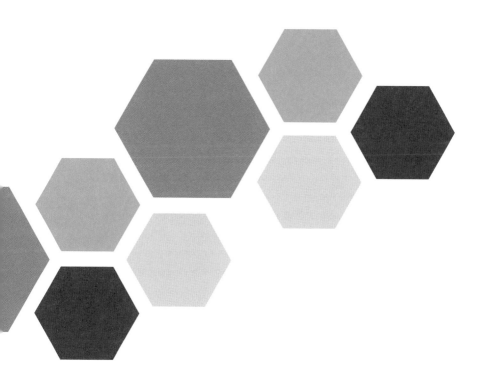

Chapter One

Why Should You Consider Starting a Provider-Sponsored Health Plan?

The world of healthcare delivery, in particular the relationship between clinical outcomes and financial reimbursement, is changing forever. Fee-for-service (FFS) medicine is being replaced by outcome-based methods that are at the heart of value-based care (or what are sometimes also called risk-based payment arrangements). At the time this book went to press in the summer of 2015, influential public and private sector payors already had committed publicly to using value-based care strategies to both lower healthcare costs and improve quality (see Figure 1.1).

> **Expert Insight**
>
> *"The insurance market is changing very quickly due to consolidation, employer forces and the expansion of narrow networks. Nearly half of health plans offered on Affordable Care Act insurance exchanges in the 2013–2014 season were narrow or ultra narrow network plans. Providers must be prepared to articulate their value to multiple audiences and for the right organization, setting up their own health plans is the ultimate expression of worth to your community."*
>
> **– Phil Kamp**
> CEO and Co-Founder, Valence Health

In the midst of this market transition, healthcare organizations and individual practitioners are still trying to understand what the transition from "volume-to-value" really means for them specifically. The market is changing quickly. Patient populations and health insurance benefits are evolving, and healthcare leaders are left wondering, "How can my organization support new care models and financial arrangements that reward improved outcomes and not just activities (i.e., value-based care)?" At the same time, healthcare providers must serve the high patient volumes associated with fee-for-service models that still dominate most parts of the country.

Government Pledges

Health and Human Services (HHS) Announcement

HHS announced goals and a timeline for shifting Medicare business to value-based care payment models (accountable care organizations (ACOs) and bundled payments):

- 30% payments by the end of 2016
- 50% payments by the end of 2018

Alliance Promises

Health Care Transformation Task Force (HCTTF)

- Several major providers and payors formed a nonprofit coalition called the HCTTF
- Each member of the HCTTF has committed to shifting 75% of its business to value-based care

Commercial Commitments

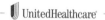

UnitedHealthcare

- Made ~$36 billion in value-based care payments in 2014
- Announced plans to increase value-based payments to providers by 20% in 2015 (more than $43 billion)

BlueCross BlueShield

- Currently pays $1 out of every $5 of medical claims to value-based programs (~$65 billion)
- Engaged with ~350 local value-based programs nationwide
- Saved ~$500 million as a result of value-based care in 2012

aetna

- Plans to increase value-based payments to be greater than one-third of total payments
- Signed 28 new contracts with ACOs in 2014
- View the government's efforts as positive, but would like to move more quickly to value-based care than HHS has committed

Source: Valence Health summary of public statements and press releases from each named organization.
Figure 1.1

Everyone agrees that the pace and complexity of change is putting stress on healthcare providers of all shapes and sizes as the benefits of value-based care models have yet to be fully realized. In order to make sound decisions that allow providers to survive and hopefully prosper, they need to understand what future services will be and how future revenues will be generated. As this shift occurs, with different nuances and at different rates across the country, providers need to be ready to invest in the critical capabilities, like new analytical skills, population health technologies and care management competencies that different value-based models demand.

While many healthcare professionals already participate in pay-for-performance contracts, a value-based care model that we at Valence Health have come to refer to as "risk-light" — the provider-sponsored health plan (PSHP) — is at the opposite end of the risk spectrum. PSHPs represent the ultimate value-based care or risk arrangement. Simply defined, a PSHP is an organization of individual practitioners, ancillary service providers and/or hospitals that come together to design and run their own

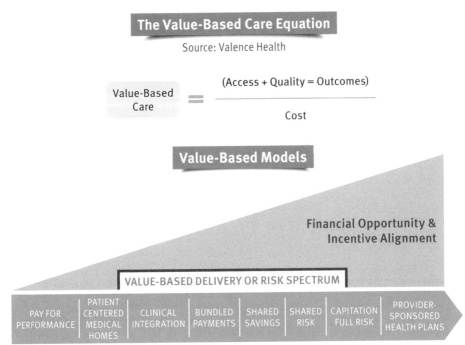

Figure 1.2

health plan (see Figure 1.2). As a result, the providers who are part of PSHPs are completely responsible for all aspects of costs, quality, network configuration, benefit design and other activities associated with providing health insurance to their members. Unlike administrators at large national or regional health plans, the administrators and owners of any PSHP are also all neighbors with the plan's members.

If healthcare providers were to make a list of things that have not worked in the past, many would say that individual providers — be they doctors or hospitals — often lack control to match meaningful quality metrics with reimbursement. Providers who are on the front lines of care delivery are the only ones who can truly manage medical costs and quality for patients. Somewhere along the line, traditional health insurers like Aetna, Cigna or one of the Blues, stopped managing insurance risk and instead started managing care. There is a big difference between underwriting a person who is in a car accident (insurance risk) versus underwriting a patient who is a chronic diabetic (medical cost management).

Providers, if responsible for patient outcomes (including the cost of delivering those outcomes), have a unique set of controls only they can execute. They are in the ideal position to help patients decide where they receive care and how often they need it; to spend time needed with a patient to confirm engagement and care compliance; or to help explain the benefits and responsibilities associated with a patient's health insurance.

The two principal goals of successful PSHP are to empower providers and capitalize on a shared mission. By bringing providers, their patients and payors closer together to create community directed health improvements (rather than paying for a certain volume of services), effective PSHPs seek to meet these goals. Of course, it takes more than just a promise of providing higher-quality care to get everyone on board, especially when that change also entails massive transformation, new investments re-training, etc. Naturally, people and the organizations they operate tend to follow the money. It is the promise of increased revenue that drives almost every industry and, clinical altruism aside, the same force also is operating in healthcare.

Historically, insurance companies have influenced a great deal of the healthcare industry. They have had the data, created the benefits or plan designs and directed medical care by providing authorizations and utilization management rules. In PSHPs, however, providers have ultimate control of driving their own "bus." To ensure that you know how your bus will operate, the rules of the road, what different routes exist and have all the necessary operating equipment, we decided to write this book, "Helping Solve the U.S. Healthcare Crisis: The Provider's Guide to Building a Successful Health Plan."

> **Expert Insight**
>
> *"The world has fundamentally changed and today, PSHPs can use data to affect outcomes and they can make it available to the doctors at point of care in order to make the right clinical decisions. I personally have always believed that the people who have the data win. Now more than ever, providers can be those winners if they are willing to accept the challenges and hard work that come with starting a PSHP."*
>
> **– R. Todd Stockard**
> President and Co-Founder, Valence Health

Of course, providers and payors are not the only stakeholders who can direct the healthcare industry. Patients, perhaps more accurately called consumers or members in health plans, are gaining increasingly more control following implementation of the Affordable Care Act (ACA) and the private sector's increased use of private exchanges. Like many industries before, the veil separating the average consumer from understanding the health plan selection process and making his or her own decision, has fallen. No matter what legislative actions are taken or Supreme Court decisions are issued in the years to come, the U.S. will very likely continue to have more and more Americans with health insurance.

Expert Insight

"We are embarking on consumerism. And those consumerism, purchasing and use behaviors are different than what the traditional model will support. That disruption in the healthcare system is where providers and provider-sponsored health plans are inserting themselves. No one goes to a travel agent anymore. There is no secret to 'I'm going to put you on this plane and book a flight' anymore."

– Daniel Yunker
CEO, Land of Lincoln Health
President and CEO, Metropolitan Chicago Healthcare Council

Now that public and private health insurance exchanges have been used, general consumer knowledge will continue to increase as patients self-educate. As more patients/consumers/members directly experience health plan shopping and value-based care, they also will want greater transparency, more information and potentially even different products and plan designs.

Expert Insight

"It's going to be like Expedia for health plans."

– Steve Cherok
Healthcare Vertical Practice Leader, Trion Group,
A Marsh & McLennan Agency, LLC Company

Perhaps the best analogy comes from the travel market. Much like the early transition to consumer-focused travel technology, the mystery and challenges associated with choosing and enrolling in a health plan are beginning to fade. There was a time — hard though it may be to remember — when we had no means of scheduling flights for ourselves, making us completely dependent on travel agents and agencies. These days, an individual can schedule a flight in a few minutes without leaving his or her chair.

Frankly, the healthcare industry is following the same route. Everyone, from the uninsured and small business owners to employees of Fortune 100 companies, has the ability to make healthcare insurance and provision decisions. And these choices only will become easier as medical terminology, quality-rating systems and the health insurance industry as a whole become more transparent. It is on this newly paved highway that providers and PSHP buses are particularly well-poised to gain significant advantages.

> **Expert Insight**
>
> *"As people begin to think differently and choose how they consume and purchase healthcare, it allows for new, innovative options to enter the marketplace. And we firmly believe that PSHPs are the best chance to truly impact population health."*
>
> **– Jason Montrie**
> President, Land of Lincoln Health

Additionally, in 2014, there was an abundance of negative news coverage about health insurance, and the bumpy start to the launch of the ACA did not help. As a result, many consumers still do not really trust large health insurance companies.

The good news is that performance ratings are more favorable than ever for community affiliated and provider-sponsored health plans. In fact, in athenahealth's 2015 Payer-View® Report™, released for the 10th consecutive year, the top two rated health insurers were nontraditional health plans. The report measures payors' financial, administrative and transactional performance, providing a snapshot of changing payor dynamics.

Out of 166 Payors, Small, Regional, Commercial Plans and Blues Plans Dominate the Top 10

Source: athenahealth

2014	2015	Payor
2	1	HealthPartners
5	2	Group Health Cooperative
1	3	Humana

- Health Partners (Nonprofit, MN) and Group Health Cooperative (Nonprofit, WA) move into winning ranks
- Humana and BCBS-MA continue to perform well and remained in the Top 10 for 2014

Figure 1.3

With advances in technology, business intelligence and information-sharing platforms, there are more tools available today to help all types of healthcare organizations design, build and successfully run a PSHP. Coupled with strong consumer support and the market's commitment to using (and in the case of Medicare, potentially mandating) value-based care arrangements, the time has never been better for organizations to consider developing their own PSHP. In the same vein, we know that becoming a PSHP is a huge undertaking. It will not and should not be the value-based care solution for everyone. However, there has never been a better time for you to figure out if running your own health plan is even a consideration.

The PSHPs' Unique Risk/Reward Equation

As with all potential ventures, there are upsides and downsides to consider. Risk defines the potential downside of any business, but the potential reward is what piques everyone's interest.

As we give you our perspectives on the key risks and rewards of PSHPs, we want to briefly discuss the differences between insurance risk and medical cost management. While there are many aspects of insurance risk — like the risk associated with underwriting a policy and setting the prices that should be charged for certain types of coverage — it also is important to mention that PSHPs can take numerous approaches to managing insurance risk. For example, there are tools like reinsurance and stop-loss coverage that are available to any health plan including PSHPs to specifically help address and mitigate insurance risks.

Medical cost management represents an organization's ability to manage groups of patients or populations and help direct their medical care in ways that will produce the most favorable health outcomes at the lowest possible costs. Here, many experts would say that PSHPs have a distinct advantage in providing medical cost management over large national insurance companies.

Since PSHPs are owned, managed and governed by providers themselves, they are uniquely qualified to determine the right level of medical management and the most appealing care delivery systems for the patients in their communities. Every healthcare system, physician group and hospital that is part of a successful PSHP will all unite around devising and refining approaches to the plan's medical cost management to lower their insurance risk. Additionally, PSHPs share a common mission as their governing members also are joined by a shared desire to improve the health and well-being of their neighbors.

Potential Risks

Let's be frank, PSHPs are not for the faint of heart and many of us remember PSHPs that failed in the 1990s. Even though times have changed, which we will detail more in Chapter 2, "How Today's PSHPs are Different," it is important to recognize that providers who successfully run PSHPs rely on extensive amounts of research, forethought, determination and outside support. Having had the opportunity to work for and alongside some very successful PSHPs, we wanted to share our insights around nine critical business questions your organization needs to honestly discuss and deeply analyze to determine if becoming PSHP is a viable option for you.

Given the significant investment of both time and money PSHPs require, it is essential to conduct a comprehensive feasibility analysis that answers tough, but real, questions. Specifically, we recommend that you:

- **Identify the potential network size and types of providers you will need:** What physicians would be participating in the plan? How strong are their primary care bases and what specialties do they offer? What percentage of a physician's patient base will likely be enrolled in your PSHP? What current or potential physician partnerships does the organization have to increase patients' in-network options? How would the PSHP's profits and losses be divided among these different entities? Who will govern these hospital and physician partnerships and their revenue?

- **Evaluate your change management capabilities:** If you need new care protocols and reimbursement models to be successful in your PSHP, is your plan's book of business big enough to get physicians to change their behaviors? Can you teach and train network members about new reimbursement models and population health management tools?

- **Analyze the organization's market position and local competition:** What is the delivery organization's market share within its respective service area? How many other competitors are within the geographic area and what degree of competitive advantage do your providers have over other local providers?

- **Assess local payor reaction:** Will independent payors still be willing to work with your organization, even if reluctantly? If not, can your providers survive without those other contracts?

> **Expert Insight**
>
> *"There is a lot of investment on behalf of payors on their network strategy; if a provider disrupts that network strategy or makes alterations to it, the payor may not be happy and could course-correct."*
>
> **– Matthew Levin**
> Executive Vice President Head of Global Strategy, Aon

- **Gauge consumers' buy-in:** How will your region's consumers and employers respond to a provider-sponsored health plan? Will the total population of potential consumers grow or shrink over time?

- **Investigate your specific regulatory environment:** What existing legislation encourages or prevents PSHPs from realizing their potential? What unique Department of Insurance regulations in your state may come into play?

- **Consider costs and financial realities:** Do you have the cash on hand and a bond rating high enough to allow it to set aside the necessary reserves? What type of stop-loss insurance do you need and what types of care spend could your PSHP live with?

Expert Insight

"Some hospitals or organizations just don't have the capital, or don't want to deploy the capital for that long of a payback into something that they are not all that familiar with doing."

– Lon Sprecher
Former President and CEO, Dean Health Plan

- **Evaluate different sales options:** Will your provider-sponsored health plan be sold to individuals or groups? Would it be more effective to sell the plan directly to consumers via exchanges? Will insurance brokers be used to sell the plan? Will the plan only serve a discrete population, such as Medicare or Medicaid, or a defined set of local employees, like a Multiple Employer Welfare Association (MEWA)?

- **Assess your insurance IQ:** Do you have, or can you recruit or partner with professionals who have the knowledge and experience to run an insurance company? Do you have resources to evaluate the statutory and federal health insurance regulations that vary by state, by payor and change over time?

Accurately and objectively analyzing these questions is crucial, not just to gauge the potential success of your PSHP, but to determine whether to ultimately move forward. The good news is that after you conduct this type of a feasibility study, you will be steeped in critical value-based care information and much more ready to take on greater amounts of risk — even if that means bundled payment and shared savings contracts. For those groups that decide to pursue PSHPs, you will also be ahead of the game and have much of the information you will need to fine-tune the engine of your PSHP's bus.

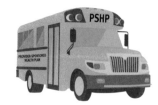

Potential Rewards

We are all well aware of some of the most successful provider-sponsored health plans, from well-known national players like Intermountain and Kaiser Permanente, to regional leaders like Driscoll Children's Health Plan in Texas and Alliant Health Plans in Dalton, Georgia. These organizations and the more than 120 PSHPs currently operating in the U.S. have shown that their plans have some distinct advantages over other types of health plans.

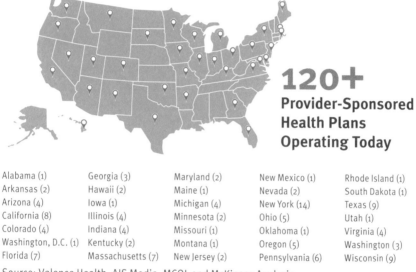

120+
Provider-Sponsored Health Plans Operating Today

Alabama (1)	Georgia (3)	Maryland (2)	New Mexico (1)	Rhode Island (1)
Arkansas (2)	Hawaii (2)	Maine (1)	Nevada (2)	South Dakota (1)
Arizona (4)	Iowa (1)	Michigan (4)	New York (14)	Texas (9)
California (8)	Illinois (4)	Minnesota (2)	Ohio (5)	Utah (1)
Colorado (4)	Indiana (4)	Missouri (1)	Oklahoma (1)	Virginia (4)
Washington, D.C. (1)	Kentucky (2)	Montana (1)	Oregon (5)	Washington (3)
Florida (7)	Massachusetts (7)	New Jersey (2)	Pennsylvania (6)	Wisconsin (9)

Source: Valence Health, AIS Media, MCOL and McKinsey Analysis

Figure 1.4

For example, PSHPs typically offer more effective and efficient population health management. Some studies suggest that PSHPs are more efficient, paving the way for the provider-sponsored payor to offer lower premiums, create additional incentives and pass savings on to their members.

Taking Control of What Really Matters

Most importantly in a PSHP, you are your own boss. Enjoy that for a moment.

When a healthcare organization and an insurance plan work together as a unified entity, it allows them to make decisions and implement initiatives that are mutually beneficial. This kind of thinking begins in your initial feasibility assessment and continues as your PSHP grows and matures.

Everyone wins by:

- Deciding the right level of risk

- Determining how to manage that risk

- Controlling when new products will be offered

- Determining how to market and deliver your products

- Deciding the clinical metrics and controls that will be used to impact both access to and payment for care

> **Expert Insight**
>
> *"From a control perspective, you are now making the rules. You are the insurance company. So things you may have perceived as burdensome to the provider, you now have more control over."*
>
> **– Lou DiGiovine**
> Vice President of Client Financial Services, Valence Health

A key determinant of the right level of risk for any PSHP can be defined by the payors and patients you choose to work with — both initially and in the long run.

Specifically, some PSHPs choose to start small and gain experience. Ultimately, different payors have different needs, so many of the strategic and tactical decisions your plan makes will be intimately tied to your plan's decision to offer commercial, Medicare and Medicaid health plans. Also remember that as a PSHP, your degree of control extends far beyond choosing which payors you will work with. Legislation surrounding health plans and health insurance changes over time, and as a PSHP, you can help influence future health insurance policymaking.

Commercial

In the commercial payor world, one deals with employment-based health insurance. Some PSHPs will choose to directly contract with self-insured employers, becoming one health plan option or the preferred health plan an employer offers to its employees. In many communities, however, a health system is also that area's largest employer. Therefore, some PSHPs are created to serve the healthcare needs of their own employees and their employees' dependents. In either example, when offering a PSHP to commercial payors, the need to deal with brokers who sell health insurance plans to employers usually becomes part of the equation. In fact, some HR professionals

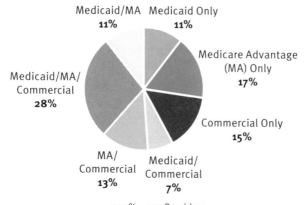

Provider Systems are Offering a Range of Health Plans

Source: 2013 AIS database; 2014 InterStudy database; CMS MA enrollment data; McKinsey analysis

- Medicaid/MA 11%
- Medicaid Only 11%
- Medicare Advantage (MA) Only 17%
- Medicaid/MA/Commercial 28%
- Commercial Only 15%
- Medicaid/Commercial 7%
- MA/Commercial 13%

100% = 107 Providers
The percentages shown do not sum to 100 because of rounding.

Figure 1.5

only consider health plans for the employees they represent — if that plan is offered by a health insurance broker (for more detailed information about insurance brokers, refer to Chapter 5, "Sales and Marketing").

Medicare

When PSHPs serve Medicare-eligible patients, there will be a number of forms, service offering and reporting guidelines that your PSHP will have to follow or comply with per the U.S. Centers for Medicare and Medicaid Services (CMS). In Medicare Advantage, the full-risk payment option available through CMS, some PSHPs will choose to directly contract with CMS. Others will accept a Medicare Advantage contract from a commercial payor, therefore becoming fully sub-capitated to a payor like Humana or Cigna. In the case of a sub-capitated Medicare Advantage arrangement, the commercial plan takes on some of the administrative duties, like paying claims and reporting to CMS. If a PSHP contracts directly with CMS, the PSHP will have to fulfill all of those responsibilities.

Medicaid

Medicaid differs dramatically from state to state and in some cases, like in California, from county to county. Therefore, when a PSHP engages in a Medicaid contract, there will be varying degrees of compliance, plan design and delivery requirements it will have to meet. In some cases, when Medicaid is the payor, the PSHP also may have to comply with additional CMS requirements (e.g., if there is a federal waiver in place directing certain aspects of Medicaid managed care delivery in that service area). In some states, Medicaid managed care members are enrolled automatically in health plans and in other states, there are choice provisions. Bottom line, you will need to know just what your state's or county's Medicaid options look like before deciding whether offering products to this payor can help your PSHP meet its business and civic objectives.

Customizable Plan Design

Large national and regional health insurance companies historically have been in control of the medical encounter and paid claims data that are used to create plan designs, which can be replicated in different geographies. With PSHPs, this equation changes as they build plans around the direct needs of their local residents. A PSHP with a connected team of actuaries and data sets can design plans using one guiding question: how can we best serve the needs of our specific populations given commercial, Medicare or Medicaid's specific requirements? You then can determine the plan's premiums and incentives to drive better behavior.

Consider that for a moment. Your PSHP will have the ability to shape patient behavior by rewarding certain actions. Do you want a specific population to see the doctor more often? Give them incentives to get preventative care. Do you want to encourage regular screenings for a common ailment in the elderly, children or expecting mothers? The key policymaking tools are at your disposal.

PSHPs also can directly influence the physicians, and other healthcare professionals and institutions that are part of the plan's network by designing and enforcing clinical quality guidelines that will both lower costs and improve care. For many providers, that is the biggest benefit to having a PSHP. PSHPs can be very successful in conducting provider and patient education and outreach that helps to keep care delivery within the PSHPs' defined networks. PSHPs know their providers personally and in some cases, those same providers are part of the PSHPs' governing structure.

Increased Consumer Access

A common mission among all healthcare institutions is to improve access to care. PSHPs — through their customizable plan designs and provider relations expertise — can expand their offerings to insure more people can access care where it is needed the most.

About 75 percent[1] of medical costs are for preventable conditions. PSHPs are ideally suited to identify these preventable conditions, offer locally tailored programs to combat them and create incentives for consumers and providers to participate. Your organization can improve patient access not only to diagnostic care, but also to preventative care.

PSHPs also tend to attract consumers who prefer to stay local. The state and federal exchanges created by the ACA have brought a new group of health insurance consumers into the market and many of these exchange members are attracted to PSHP products.

The ACA also funded 27 brand new health consumer-operated-and-oriented plans (CO-OPs). While CO-OPs are not PSHPs, they share a similar mission around improving community health and wellness at more reasonable costs. They also tend to work very collaboratively with their provider communities to make decisions around critical plan-related things like benefit design and care coordination rules. While CO-OPs were only 18 months old at the time of this book's publication, they have shown great commitment in structuring their relationships with providers to use value-based care reimbursement models in ways that are very similar to PSHPs.

Economics

> **Expert Insight**
>
> *"From a financial perspective, it makes sense: you are controlling the premium. The premium is coming in, and in a traditional health plan, that is an expense. For PSHPs, it is an expense also, but in the consolidation, it is a part of revenue. So from that perspective, it is giving the provider much more control of the premium dollars that are coming in. That is a huge driver on why an organization would want to start a PSHP."*
>
> **– Lon Sprecher**
> Former President and CEO, Dean Health Plan

In PSHPs and any value-based care arrangement, you want inpatient reimbursement to drop as a result of lower hospital and emergency room utilization. Experts

---

1 1) Institute of Medicine reports 2) New England Journal of Medicine 3) Centers for Disease Control 4) Richard Clarke, Wall Street Journal 5) Commonwealth Fund

agree that one of the keys to remaining successful in PSHPs and value-based care is cutting unnecessary costs from the care delivery process and shifting revenue to other settings.

> **Expert Insight**
>
> *"If you are contracted with a commercial insurance company, you're exporting 70 cents out of every $1 you save to that other company. Whereas, if you have a provider-owned health plan, you are in a closed circle for at least the members who come through with the health plan, and you are saving 100% of every $1 that you are taking out of the system."*
>
> **– Lon Sprecher**
> Former President and CEO, Dean Health Plan

On the cost-cutting side, provider-sponsored health plans also eliminate the administrative middleman, making them no longer dependent on an entity that is far removed from actual care provision. PSHPs can design their own, more efficient and cost-effective administrative tools. Research conducted by the Urban Institute and the Sherlock Company shows that independent PSHPs have more efficient and less costly administrative operations — making them a better value for payors.[2]

Instead of sending a large portion of every dollar saved into another insurance company's bank account, a PSHP can keep the majority of every dollar within its own system. It also can use those dollars in ways that make sense for the community the PSHP serves. On top of this, PSHPs provide an alternative revenue stream that extends beyond "old-fashioned" hospital-based inpatient care.

Value-based care and population health management strategies used by PSHPs are more heavily focused on shifting revenue to the front or start of the care system. Building out a clinically integrated primary care and specialty network and driving revenue and patient care to it needs to overtake the volume-based revenue model that many hospitals still employ.

In some successful PSHPs, both hospitals and the plan share the same balance sheet; therefore, in the big picture, the PSHP business is counter-cyclical to the hospital's business. From an economic standpoint, your health plan can be a hedg-

---

2 Berenson, Robert and Coughlin, Teresa. "Success Factors in Five High-Quality, Low-Cost Health Plans." Sherlock, Douglas B. CFA, Sherlock Company webinar presentation, July 2014.

ing or diversification play, meaning when inpatient revenues are down, health plan revenue can be up.

Improving Quality of Care

Value, as defined by the patient, is a core element of delivering quality care. This value can be found through the individual member experience or on a larger scale, with a connected, integrated healthcare community. Be careful to never discount the importance of a connected healthcare environment in creating value.

When you manage your own health plan, you gain more control over the quality of your connected healthcare environment. For example, as a PSHP, you can make benefit and operating decisions such that when elderly patients are discharged from an inpatient hospital stay, home health services are available to appropriately keep these patients in their own homes rather than in a skilled nursing facility. It is your organization that helps develop the provider network by bringing in good providers, while eliminating the bad. By narrowing the scope of your network to only exceptional providers, you can improve care coordination among more patients. You also can increase member retention by incentivizing the providers and patients who stay in your network to reinforce these quality guidelines.

Likewise, quality can be compromised by the predictable variation in physicians' style of care delivery. When you add in the fact that physicians who fear malpractice liability tend to perform more defensive medicine, you can see over-utilization and inefficient use of resources, like ordering unnecessary and expensive tests. In fact, national studies routinely estimate that 30 percent to 40 percent of all medical expenses are unnecessary.[3] PSHPs aim to reduce these practices by integrating health professionals more thoroughly in the health plan's decision-making processes that authorize services and use of resources. By involving the provider community intimately in its design work, PSHPs have the opportunity to leverage evidence-based protocols and incentives at the front of care delivery systems. ⊘

---

3 1) Institute of Medicine reports 2) New England Journal of Medicine 3) Centers for Disease Control 4) Richard Clarke, Wall Street Journal 5) Commonwealth Fund

Industry Terminology Related to Why Should You Consider Starting a Provider-Sponsored Health Plan?

Commercial Health Insurance   Any type of health benefit not obtained from Medicare or Medicaid. The insurance may be employer-sponsored or privately purchased. Commercial health insurance may be provided on a fee-for-service basis or through a managed care plan.

Source: ForwardHealth.WI.gov

Health CO-OP (Consumer-operated-and-oriented plans)   Enabled by low-interest loans in the ACA, health insurance CO-OPs are private, nonprofit and member governed health insurance companies selling policies on their states' marketplaces. CO-OPs' member-oriented focus means that any surplus earned must be applied to either lowering premiums or increasing benefits.

Source: National Alliance of State Health CO-OPs, NASHCO.org

Medicaid   A state-administered health insurance program for low-income families and children, pregnant women, the elderly, people with disabilities, and in some states, other adults. The federal government provides a portion of the funding for Medicaid and sets guidelines for the program.

Source: HealthCare.gov

Medicare   A federal health insurance program for people who are age 65 or older and certain younger people with disabilities. It also covers people with End-Stage Renal Disease (permanent kidney failure requiring dialysis or a transplant, sometimes called ESRD).

Source: HealthCare.gov

Medicare Advantage   A type of Medicare health plan offered by a private company that contracts with Medicare to provide you with all your Part A and Part B benefits. Medicare Advantage plans include HMOs, PPOs, private FFS plans, Special Needs Plans and Medicare Medical Savings Account Plans. Most Medicare Advantage plans offer prescription drug coverage.

Source: HealthCare.gov

Medical Management   An umbrella term that includes utilization management, case management and disease management functions. Medical management strategies and programs are designed to improve population health by guiding consumer and/or provider behavior toward the healthiest options. Also synonymous with Medical Cost Management.

Source: Valence Health

Multiple Employer Welfare Association (MEWA)   A group of employers who join to purchase group health insurance, often self-funded to avoid state mandates and insurance regulation. By virtue of ERISA (Employee Retirement Income Security Act), such entities are little regulated, if at all. Many MEWAs have enabled small employers to obtain cost-effective health coverage, while some MEWAs have not had the financial resources to withstand the risk of medical costs and have failed.

Source: Segen's Medical Dictionary

Premium   The amount that must be paid by the insured for his/her health insurance or plan. The member or his/her employers usually pay the premium monthly, quarterly or yearly.

Source: HealthCare.gov

Reinsurance   A reimbursement system that protects insurers from very high claims. It usually involves a third party paying part of an insurance company's claims once they pass a certain amount. Reinsurance is a way to stabilize an insurance market and make coverage more available and affordable.

Source: HealthCare.gov

Stop-Loss Premium   The dollar amount of claims filed for eligible expenses at which point you have paid 100% of your out-of-pocket and the insurance begins to pay at 100%. Stop-loss is reached when an insured individual has paid the deductible and reached the out-of-pocket maximum amount of coinsurance.

Source: Healthinsurance.org

Sub-capitation   For sub-capitation agreements, the plan must provide additional payments to providers to ensure that every unit of primary care services is reimbursed at the increased rate. Plans must remove the risk to primary care providers of insufficient payments due to increased utilization.

Source: Oregon.gov

Chapter Two

How Today's PSHPs are Different

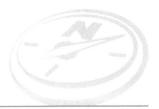

Provider-sponsored health plans (PSHPs) are not new. As you begin considering the risks and rewards associated with managing your own plan, you may be thinking, "Hey, this sounds a lot like what we tried and quite frankly failed to do with health maintenance organizations (HMOs) in the 1990s." Or you may be thinking, "I know there were a number of provider organizations that also formed health plans around that time and some failed." While both statements are true, the most critical thing to remember is that the larger healthcare ecosystem has changed dramatically.

Five Important Factors that Distinguish Today's PSHPs From the HMOs of the Past and Make for Greater Potential for Success

Source: Valence Health

1. An increased focus on quality of care
2. The availability of more data and technology to make key health plan decisions and operational course corrections
3. Increased levels of direct patient participation in their health plan purchasing decisions
4. Better price and quality transparency
5. Center for Medicare & Medicaid Services' (CMS) ever-growing preference for value-based reimbursements models that PSHPs can uniquely deliver

Figure 2.1

As discussed in Chapter 1, "Why Should You Consider Starting a Provider-Sponsored Health Plan?" there is more interest in value-based care than ever before. As the U.S. healthcare system increasingly ties reimbursement to quality, there is an equally important difference from what was done in the 1990s. One reason HMOs of the past eventually fell out of favor was due in large part to their limiting the use of healthcare services through "gatekeeper" approaches. In contrast, today's provider-sponsored health plans are not focused on imposing across-the-board limitations on utilization.

Instead, the focus is on preventative care, and identifying and encouraging access to the most effective interventions for a given condition, while identifying and discouraging access to the least effective interventions. The PSHPs we have had the privilege to work with usually build their plans around smaller, more limited networks of providers so that they can more closely coordinate care within and across those networks.

 It's not utilization management, it's population health management."

– Phil Kamp
CEO and Co-Founder, Valence Health

Knowledge is Power: Leveraging Data/Analytics

Perhaps the most important factor that makes the PSHP model more viable today is providers' greater access to data and technology. In the 1990s, healthcare providers were at a disadvantage relative to insurers. First of all, providers simply did not have access to clinical and financial data about the populations they were taking responsibility for. Second, many of the powerful technologies to perform in-depth data mining and predictive analytics were not yet available. Also, many of the PSHPs that failed in the 1990s often did not know when they were in financial trouble and did not have the chance to course-correct.

Today, in contrast, providers can choose from a variety of technologies and data sets to both build insurance products and asses their performance in meeting clinical guidelines and financial performance metrics associated with those products. In an increasing number of cases, providers have more impactful real-time information than insurers or at least are equalizing the playing field. The exciting thing about starting a PSHP now is that a wider variety of tools and services are available that enable providers to shape their own destinies.

 Today, PSHPs can use data to affect outcomes and they can make it available to the doctors at point of care in order to make the right clinical decisions. I personally have always believed that the people who have the data win."

– R. Todd Stockard
President and Co-Founder, Valence Health

Advances in big data technology and predictive modeling have evolved to a point where providers themselves can independently apply proven actuarial analysis without the help or involvement of traditional insurance companies. This visibility into financial risk and the ability to account for it are now accessible to successful provider organizations for both running their PSHPs and any other risk arrangements they take on.

As we move more deeply into value-based care, providers will likely manage a portfolio of risk arrangements. For example, a PSHP may have a shared-savings contract with its state Medicaid agency and sell several health plan products to employees who buy commercial health plans on a private exchange. Therefore, PSHPs will further need to leverage data and analytics to make sure they are diversifying their health plan product portfolios in ways that will benefit their communities and their balance sheets. Because PSHPs are smaller and in many cases more nimble than large national or regional health insurance companies, they can be much better positioned to use data and analytics to design and deliver new and more innovative health plan products and value-based reimbursement models.

Increased Patient Participation in Health Insurance Decision Making

The Affordable Care Act's (ACA) creation of public exchanges has allowed tens of millions of newly insured individuals to shop for and buy healthcare insurance. In the private healthcare marketplace, the costs of employee healthcare have gone through the roof. In 2003, it cost employers $12,400 per year on average to insure one employee and their dependents. A decade later, those costs have almost doubled. As a result, many employers have embraced value-based payments and are open to contracting directly with PSHPs in an effort to further control costs and reduce employees' out-of-pocket expenses. Alternately, other employers are now having their employees purchase healthcare insurance on private exchanges.

As a result of both exchange movements — public and private — more and more insured individuals are buying their own insurance and to date, they tend to favor narrow network products. These narrow network health plans simply limit the doctors and hospitals that members can visit. Go to doctor A or hospital A and the insurance company will pay most, if not all, of the bill. Go to doctor B or hospital B and the health plan will pay nothing or a very small part of the bill.

While a large part of narrow network health plans' popularity comes from these plans' lower prices, they also often tend to utilize a network of community providers that already have strong and positive brand recognition among consumers. PSHPs are ideally suited to offer narrow network products that address the desire for community based plans that appeal to both public and private exchange shoppers alike. Individual exchange shoppers, unlike large corporate HR buyers of health insurance, also like to buy local since they are only covering themselves and their family members. They do not typically have to worry about covering cousins in 17 other states. Therefore, locally administered and delivered PSHPs have advantages on the public and private exchanges.

Better Price and Quality Transparency

Even though people criticized HMOs in the 1990s for lack of choice, consumers today are willing to forgo broad choice if they believe their providers offer higher-quality care. When making the quality versus quantity decision, today's consumers typically take two routes: they either have an existing relationship with high-quality providers who are already part of a network they can access, or they believe their network — no matter how narrow — has a stronger reputation for delivering exceptional care.

Provider-Led Plans are Five-Star Medicare Advantage Winners

Source: Valence Health

Nine out of the 13 Five-Star Medicare Advantage Plans are Provider-Sponsored Health Plans (PSHP)

Five-Star MA Plans with Prescription Drug Coverage

- Kaiser Foundation HP, Inc.–PSHP
- Kaiser Foundation HP, of CO–PSHP
- CarePlus HP Inc.
- Kaiser Foundation HP, Inc.–PSHP
- Kaiser Foundation HP of the Mid-Atlantic States, –PSHP
- Group health Cooperative
- Gundersen HP–PSHP
- Martin's Point Gernerations, LLC
- Healthspan Integrated Care
- Kaiser Foundation HP of the NW–PSHP
- Providence HP–PSHP

Five-Star MA-Only Plans

- Medical Associates HP–PSHP
- Dean HP–PSHP

Figure 2.2

Think of it this way: if a PSHP is a "bus" it may have a route with a limited number of stops, but people are willing to walk a few extra blocks after they get off because the bus ride is so much more pleasant. For example, your potential members may be much happier picking from a specific number of providers at Intermountain Healthcare than having their choice of physicians from a number of smaller hospitals they have never heard of. If we use the Medicare Advantage Star Rating System as a proxy for consumer-quality ratings, consumers 65 years and older clearly think PSHPs are the highest-quality plans available (see Figure 2.2). As exchanges also help to make price and more quality data available, PSHPs have the opportunity to lead the way.

Centers for Medicare & Medicaid Services (CMS) and Other Recent Regulations Favor PSHPs

The country's two largest healthcare payors and regulators, Medicare and Medicaid, are highly supportive of provider-run value-based care organizations and PSHPs. Medicare Advantage (MA) specifically puts providers at full-risk for the MA members who enroll in their plans. For providers who have MA contracts, either with CMS directly or in partnership with an insurer like Humana, becoming a PSHP is a very logical next step. Medicaid also has expanded its managed care footprint across the country and many states are putting both new populations and services into their Medicaid managed care models. For example, aged, blind and disabled Medicaid recipients are now being added to Medicaid managed care programs and services like behavioral health are being added to the comprehensive offerings that Medicaid managed care programs must provide.

Additionally, many of the state and local laws that once prevented providers from gaining insurance licenses have gone away or have faced limited to no opposition when introduced. The fear that providers would somehow game the system if they were put in charge of health insurance simply has not played out. While fraud and abuse are an unfortunate part of the healthcare world, the reality is these destructive behaviors often find more fertile ground in fee-for-service models. With PSHPs, we have seen a shared commitment to improve provider quality and eliminate providers who do not practice ethical medicine.

Embracing PSHPs' Unique Differences

Some of the PSHPs that failed in the 1990s tried too hard to look and operate like large national or regional health insurance companies. Quite frankly, they failed to embrace what we have come to see as the unique benefits that PSHPs bring to their members, affiliated providers and communities.

First of all, provider-sponsored health plans have the unique advantage of being united by a mission that eludes traditional insurers: to become more fully integrated into the communities they serve by providing medical care, high-quality affordable health insurance, employment, education and more. PSHPs also have a shared commitment to improving the health and well-being of their members, who also happen to be their neighbors.

Additionally, PSHPs offer:

- **More effective population health management:** Provider-sponsored health plan leaders have firsthand knowledge of their community's healthcare needs and preferences, giving them an advantage in designing plans that deliver more customized local care. Critical decisions around what care to provide and what amount to charge for this care are both under the PSHP's control. With more tightly integrated clinical and financial performance data and metrics, PSHPs are better positioned than traditional insurers to improve outcomes and lower costs with respect to specific patient populations.

- **Higher financial reward:** Providers who offer health plans are often in the best position to benefit from first-dollar capture. Since a certain amount of inpatient costs are fixed — beds, facilities and staff — costs of incremental care often are less for a provider organization than for a traditional payor.

  For example, an episode of care might cost a traditional insurer $50,000. However, a health system sustains out-of-pocket costs that are limited to the variable costs associated with providing that care. In many instances, the variable cost of care often is less than 30 percent of the total amount billed to an insurer.

  Furthermore, up to 15 percent of an insurance company's costs are administrative. While all health insurance companies are reimbursed for their administrative costs, in a PSHP those administrative dollars stay with the organization. PSHPs can take the administrative dollars it would have paid to a traditional insurance company and reinvest that money into things like case management programs that will improve outcomes and further reduce costs. Additionally, if your PSHP is more efficient, it can choose to offer lower premiums, create additional incentives or even pass savings onto its members.

- **Greater network control:** When patients see physicians that are outside of their plan's network, it often is because their choice of doctors (or the primary care physician's referral) is outside the health plan's network of providers. Given a PSHP's long-standing relationship with its physician community, PSHPs are often much more successful in changing provider behavior. In the case of referrals, PSHPs can clearly play a much stronger role in encouraging primary care physicians to issue referrals for healthcare services within the same system. This can help improve care coordination and promote patient-centered care, while still satisfying patient preferences and health needs within the network. With more patients staying inside the PSHP's network, the member health systems can also improve market share and remain competitive.

Today's PSHPs Deliver More Meaningful Incentives

Another major distinction between HMOs of the past and PSHPs is who is driving the bus. A PSHP puts providers in the driver's seat with full control of providing care to the plan's patient population. Since doctors and other healthcare practitioners interact with these patients every day, PSHP practitioners understand community health issues, allowing them to be better prepared for and respond more quickly to changes in population health.

> *If your physicians aren't engaged (in your PSHP) and don't believe in what you're doing and they're not communicating with you, you won't make it. You just can't do it. I've been heartened by the fact that Sutter Health as an organization has relationships with 5,000 physicians who get it and want to be part of the change. They understand that it means sacrifice on their part as well as an opportunity to advance the community interests that we serve."*
>
> **– Stephen Nolte**
> CEO, Sutter Health Plus

While it is true that PSHPs and the HMOs of the 1990s both use per-member-per-month (PMPM) reimbursement methodologies, there are important differences. In the 1990s, in addition to PMPM reimbursement, primary care capitation also was at play. This meant physicians had to limit the type and amount of primary care services they could deliver to patients who had been assigned to them. The result was a set of disincentives that caused some doctors to fill their practice with fee-for-service (FFS) patients. By seeing more FFS patients, physicians received additional money on top of the capitated payments they were receiving for their HMO members. This made it harder for HMO patients to make appointments and when these HMO patients finally were able to get in to see their physicians, they were often frustrated by the poor customer service and long wait times.

While the "money first" approach attributed to HMOs may have saved money in the short term, it also led to care issues in the long run. Consider a bus that transports its passengers to their destinations quickly, but is in poor condition and its driver does not follow the rules of the road. Certainly, the bus owner is saving money on repairs and fuel, but the quality of the riders' experience was awful, causing them to seek alternative modes of transportation.

This just is not the case with today's PSHPs. While PMPM payments are alive and well, you find that PSHPs often use creative incentive programs to bring added value to practitioners who provide preventative care and improve health outcomes. It also is common to have PSHPs tie a portion of any PMPM payment to providers' abilities to meet certain quality metrics. These types of arrangements clearly incent physicians to appropriately and effectively manage patient care, while also providing more efficient non-redundant services.

> **Expert Insight**
>
> *"The rest of the world is catching up to the Kaiser/Dean/Geisinger model, which is having the doctors in control of providing care to the patient and not the bureaucratic chief medical officers from a national plan.*
>
> *Everything that you try to do is based on higher quality at lower costs and patient experience. The old triple aim."*
>
> **– Lon Sprecher**
> Former President and CEO, Dean Health Plan

Lastly, the industry as a whole has come to recognize that sicker people need more care. Therefore, we now have risk-adjusted PMPM models, so as a health plan, you can now pay providers more money if their attributed population is sicker.

Bottom line, today there are a set of forces at play that have fundamentally changed how providers can take control of the care they provide both clinically as well as financially.

With HMOs of the 1990s, providers were basically paid on an age and sex basis. For example, Medicare would historically pay a set rate for all females age 70 to 74 in a certain market.

That per-member-per-month rate was the total spend divided by the number of females in that group–that was it. If a provider got proportionately sicker patients in this group, that provider would lose money."

– R. Todd Stockard
President and Co-Founder, Valence Health

Joining the PSHP Hall of Fame

It is important to note that the health plans like Geisinger, Intermountain, Health-Partners, Alliant and Dean all were operating at the same time as many of the unsuccessful HMOs or PSHPs of the 1990s. Yet these aforementioned organizations did not get the same "bad rap" or negative attention that the unsuccessful HMOs or PSHPs of the 1990s were saddled with. These same plans are regularly held up as examples of how the healthcare system can and should work as they typically achieve better health outcomes, are able to coordinate care in a more cost-effective manner and have more satisfied members. Also, their creative execution strategies and tactics helped them survive the financial perils that befell some of their comrades in the 1990s. A perfect example of one such successful and often unsung PSHP is Driscoll Health Plan, which has marketed itself as Medicaid-centric plan for almost 20 years.

The Case for Driscoll

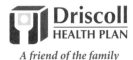

Licensed by the state of Texas as a health maintenance organization (HMO) in 1998, Driscoll Health Plan is a non-profit community-based health insurance plan that operates in south Texas. It is affiliated with Driscoll Children's Hospital, a south Texas institution that has operated for decades. For many consumers in areas like Corpus Christi, Driscoll is the best children's hospital, though it certainly helps that it is the only children's hospital in the area. After Driscoll, the nearest children's hospital is some 200 miles away in Houston. Driscoll provides other community services and is one of the area's largest employers. As a result, Driscoll has become a renowned institution for families in south Texas and is trusted by the community.

In the mid-to-late 1990s, Congress expanded Medicaid eligibility to include a greater number of people with disabilities, children, pregnant women and the elderly. Part of this expansion was the creation of the Children's Health Insurance Program (CHIP). When the state of Texas enacted the CHIP program, it also required these new enrollees to use Medicaid managed care organizations for their care.

Driscoll seized upon this opportunity and the organization decided to start a health plan for CHIP members, anticipating the state would eventually mandate Medicaid managed care coverage for the Temporary Assistance for Needy Families' (TANF) populations at some point in the future. Strategically, Driscoll also wanted to take the opportunity to help decrease the number of uninsured children in south Texas and have greater control over the per-member-per-month (PMPM) dollars that would be paid to each managed care organization. It also knew that if it did not move fast to establish itself in south Texas, it would soon face stiff competition from large for-profit Medicaid health plans. Therefore, Driscoll took action to win over some of the market and differentiate its plan on the quality of care delivered to its members.

In 2006, when the state of Texas finally mandated Medicaid managed care coverage for the TANF population in the Nueces Service Area (14 counties), it awarded the opportunity to cover the south Texas population to Driscoll and two other organizations. The newly enrolled TANF population had the choice of enrolling with one of three authorized Medicaid managed care organizations. Still hoping to get more lives under its care, Driscoll followed the Medicaid marketing regulations and used grassroots efforts to promote the Driscoll Health Plan. In the end, since the community knew and trusted Driscoll, two-thirds of the newly eligible TANF population that enrolled in a plan chose to enroll in the Driscoll plan.

Driscoll leveraged its local community ties, brand recognition and support from providers within its community to gain a strong foothold in the market. As a result, enrollment in Driscoll's Health Plan rocketed from 11,000 to 50,000 members almost overnight. By being the first and only PSHP in a market that was not dominated by a national insurer or HMO, and focusing on a potential member community that trusted the organization, Driscoll Health Plan achieved remarkable success.

Another particularly big facet of Driscoll's success was its partnership with a group of experienced provider-sponsored health plan (PSHP) professionals. Though it originally began working with a local third-party administrative firm in the late 1990s, Driscoll transitioned to working with Valence Health in the early 2000s, as it felt Valence Health could better help it reach its goals of serving a larger number of members. By improving customer service and claims administration and management, and other areas, Valence Health allowed Driscoll the opportunity to help it become an organization capable of taking on the majority of the market by not diverting energy in the "back office" process.

Today, Driscoll Health Plan cares for more than 140,000 members. As part of its longer-term strategy, the health plan has remained connected to the children's hospital and always has had a separate executive team. The two organizations have separate boards, but share some common members and are able to look at consolidated financial statements. Therefore, both the health plan and the health system know only too well that there have been years when the plan produced margin for the system and other years when the plan was supported financially by the system. In their shared commitment to improving the health of children and families in south Texas, both the health plan and the hospital are committed to improving population health.

Perhaps one of Driscoll Health Plan's greatest achievements has been the amazing community partnerships it has formed to carry out this mission. As a children's hospital, Driscoll did not deliver babies; therefore, when Driscoll Health Plan got started, it did not have any relationships with obstetricians and gynecologists. Over the years, it has formed a set of high-quality affiliations, developed case management programs and devised Medicaid-approved patient and provider incentives to reduce premature births in an extremely high-risk patient population. The Driscoll Health System also hired four maternal-fetal medicine specialists to fill a void in south Texas for pregnant women, with the desire to provide more sophisticated management of high-risk pregnancies. Driscoll Health Plan also started the Cadena de Madres (Chain of Mothers) program to provide prenatal education, lactation consulting and nutritional counseling to pregnant women enrolled in the State of Texas Access Reform program. With these programs in place, premature births have dropped 34 percent.

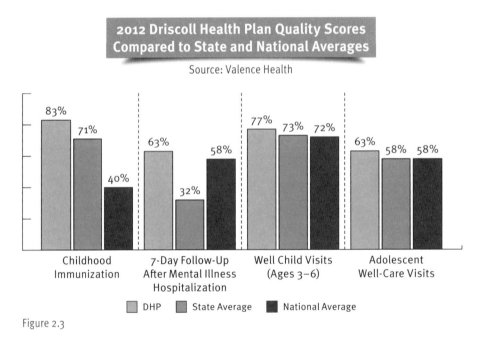

Figure 2.3

As Dr. Mary Dale Peterson shared at the second annual Valence Heath Pediatric Collaborative, "We know our entire community will be better off if the health plan and all the providers in south Texas work to reduce Neonatal Intensive Care Unit Days. Healthy babies have a much great chance of being healthy children. In the end, that is a goal that can bring us closer together, and allows us to rally around the same quality goals and incentive structures."

Using What Driscoll and Others Can Teach Us About Value-Based Care

We know from 20 years of t providers to design, build and run value-based care arrangements, that operating a PSHP is very different from running a hospital, a health system or a large physician group. There are new processes, competencies and skills that you and your organization will need to learn or acquire. In fact, we have said for years that given our wonderful work with so many provider organizations, that we should write a book. So we have done just that. In our opinion, the environment for PSHPs has never been more favorable. You do not have to go it alone; in fact, you are in great company. As you consider your options, we have taken the time to outline the basics of becoming a PSHP so you can evaluate your readiness. We really do believe it is the ultimate value-based care bus ride. ⊘

Industry Terminology Related to How Today's PSHPs are Different

Capitation   A specified amount of money paid to a health plan or doctor. This is used to cover the cost of a health plan member's healthcare services for a certain length of time.

Source: CMS.gov

Gated and Ungated Care   In the insurance industry, "gated" generically describes a plan that requires a referral from a primary care physician before a patient can visit a specialist. The doctor, his/her staff and the insurance company are positioned as gatekeepers to eliminate unnecessary testing and procedures. The cost of gated health insurance plans is less than non-gated plans, ones that allow customers to freely seek services from a specialist. Non-gated health insurance policies are more flexible, and as such usually demand higher premiums.

Source: eHow.com

Health Maintenance Organization (HMO)   A type of health insurance plan that usually limits coverage to care from doctors who work for or contract with the HMO. It generally will not cover out-of-network care except in an emergency. An HMO may require you to live or work in its service area to be eligible for coverage. HMOs often provide integrated care and focus on prevention and wellness.

Source: HealthCare.gov

Medicaid   A state-administered health insurance program for low-income families and children, pregnant women, the elderly, people with disabilities, and in some states, other adults. The federal government provides a portion of the funding for Medicaid and sets guidelines for the program.

Source: HealthCare.gov

Medicare   A federal health insurance program for people who are age 65 or older and certain younger people with disabilities. It also covers people with End-Stage Renal Disease (permanent kidney failure requiring dialysis or a transplant, sometimes called ESRD).

Source: HealthCare.gov

Medicare Advantage   A type of Medicare health plan offered by a private company that contracts with Medicare to provide you with all your Part A and Part B benefits. Medicare Advantage plans include HMOs, PPOs, private FFS plans, Special Needs Plans and Medicare Medical Savings Account Plans. Most Medicare Advantage plans offer prescription drug coverage.

Source: HealthCare.gov

Medicare Advantage Star Rating System   Medicare uses a Star Rating System to measure how well Medicare Advantage and prescription drug (Part D) plans perform. Medicare scores how well plans did in several categories, including quality of care and customer service. The overall star rating score provides a way to compare performance among several plans.

Source: MedicareInteractive.org

Narrow Network Health Plan   Limits providers to a select group to make costs more affordable to members.

Source: NYTimes.com

Per-Member-Per-Month (PMPM)   Refers to the ratio of a service or cost divided by the number of members in a group. For example, if 10,000 members of an HMO had $20,000 in spending for cardiovascular surgery, the cost per member would be $2 per month.

Source: American Academy of Family Physicians

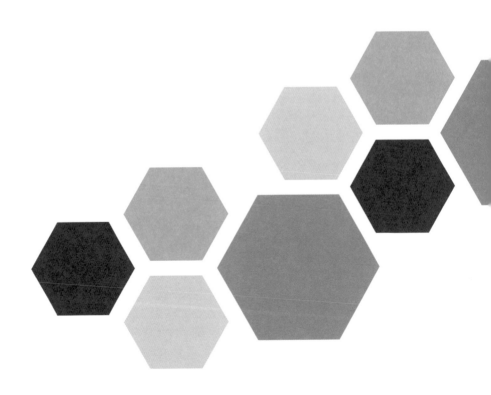

Part Two
HOW TO BECOME A PSHP

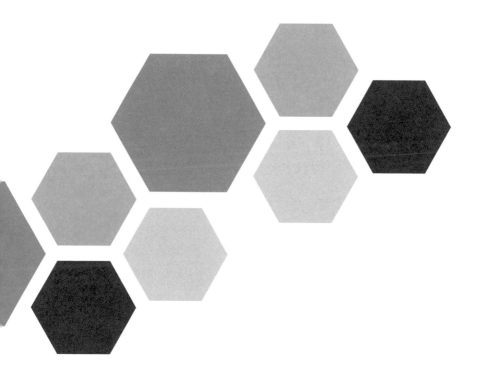

Chapter Three

Determining Your PSHP's Comprehensive Execution Strategy

The healthcare industry is far from stagnant. With the implementation of the Affordable Care Act (ACA) in 2014 and the numerous government and commercial payors that have committed to using value-based care models to transform clinical and financial outcomes and metrics, individual providers and provider organizations are rapidly performing tune-ups to ensure their care delivery vehicles are optimized.

At this very unique point in time, the decision to become a provider-sponsored health plan (PSHP) offers you the freedom to either follow the more traditional road for providing health insurance or to break from current paradigms and create an entirely new route. The ability to reinvent the wheel — or the whole bus — will be intertwined and impacted by your comprehensive execution strategy decisions.

Crafting Your PSHP's Value Proposition

Before embarking on the development of a health plan that will dramatically change your healthcare organization or medical group, it is important for your team to answer this question: Why should **our** PSHP exist?

This seemingly simple question is essential because the answer should constantly guide your health plan's creation process. Whatever your answer may be, by making it a guiding principle (see Figure 3.1) throughout the work that lies ahead, you are assured to end up with a unified business strategy. From our more than 20 years helping design, build and run PSHPs, we also have seen that failed provider-sponsored health plans either lacked agreement on the answer to this key question, or did not make execution decisions that fully supported their value proposition.

As with any business, a consumer has multiple products to choose from at a variety of different price points. So to distinguish your plan from the rest, you must develop your own unique value proposition. To put it more bluntly: Where does your PSHP fit in the healthcare ecosystem? What can it do *better* or *differently* than anyone else?

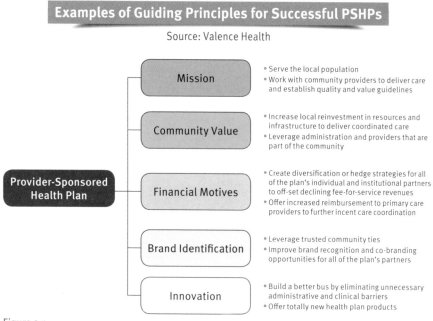

Figure 3.1

If you can pinpoint — and then sell and deliver on — the answer to this question, you are well on your way to ensuring the success of your PSHP. Using this knowledge as the cornerstone of your business model will allow you to tailor products that will help you outsell your competition. But before you can start designing a health plan (refer to Chapter 4, "Plan Design"), you absolutely have to agree on what your PSHP's guiding principle will be.

At the same time as you gain this consensus, it also is essential to conduct market research and perform a capability assessment to evaluate your organization's core competencies. The information that is gathered during these efforts — and its constant reevaluation in the upcoming years — is critical when making execution strategy decisions for your PSHP.

PSHP Market Research and Capability Assessments

Your market potential ultimately defines the parameters of your product's reach. Each factor can expand or contract your market potential and will change over time. By critically assessing each factor, your organization can mold its PSHP business model to serve those areas of the local market that present the best opportunities for you.

Key Factors Impacting PSHPs' Ability to Gain Market Share

Source: Valence Health

- Payor competition and concentration
- Provider competition
- Available consumers/members

Figure 3.2

Understanding Payor Competition and Concentration

Welcome to the insurance industry! You are already familiar with the big payors in your area, as you have negotiated contracts with and accepted fee-for-service reimbursements from them for years. In some markets, there may also be some unique payors that you will also have to consider (see Figure 3.3). As a PSHP, you will now be competing against them.

To be the best competitor you can be, you need market research to really understand each competitor insurance company's local market share. Thankfully, there are relatively straightforward ways to do this. The National Association of Insurance Commissioners (NAIC) mandates that all insurance organizations report their financial statements. This gives the NAIC a wealth of information, including each insurance company's revenue, medical costs, administrative costs and average number of members.

Health insurance is licensed at the state level, so your state's insurance regulator or agency may have valuable data that you can access to create a better understanding of your payor competition. Lastly, if there is a state or federal healthcare insurance marketplace in your community, data about who is offering what and to whom also can help you understand what other plans (buses) are driving around on your local highways. In some areas of the country, no one payor holds a strong competitive advantage, while other regions contain a major payor that dominates the market.

In addition to understanding general market share information of other health insurance companies in your area, you really need to understand these companies' market share by their major lines of health insurance business: commercial, Medicare and Medicaid.

In this more narrow sense, your PSHP may be able to fill an unmet market need. For example, in the commercially focused world of employer and individually funded health

Other Less Well-Known Health Insurance Lines of Business in the U.S.

Source: Valence Health

- Federal Employees Health Benefits Program
- Indian Health Service
- Veterans Health Administration
- Military Health System/TRICARE
- Union-Sponsored Health Benefits Programs

Figure 3.3

insurance, there may be groups of similar employers that are dissatisfied with their health insurance options. Therefore, your PSHP may be able to design offerings that are ideally suited for the small group market, creating a distinct opportunity for you.

Alternatively, if the states in your intended service area expand Medicaid and/or move to a Medicaid managed care (MMC) delivery system, your PSHP may be ideally positioned to serve that market. While many providers may have previously dismissed Medicaid as having less-than-desirable reimbursement rates, remember that as a PSHP, you take fee-for-service out of the equation.

Another way to narrow in on the types of products your PSHP should offer is to research and be aware of different concentration levels (see Figure 3.4) in your community that will impact your PSHP's business line selections.

Finally, as you develop an understanding of your health insurance market, it is equally important to have an understanding of what different payors' market shares are at the institutional and individual practitioner level. This information will give you valuable insight into your PSHP's ability to ultimately attract both patients and providers to be part of your plan's network as well.

For example, if you can attract more members to join your PSHP who are likely to have their first child in next two years, you may have a greater ability to form partnerships with obstetricians, gynecologists and pediatricians. If you then know what share of an individual physician's revenue your PSHP contributes, you also can get a sense for how much influence your PSHP will likely have in changing care practices among certain providers. Take the case where your PSHP represents 5 percent of the dollars that come into the practice. If you want to change how that group treats patients, you will likely have less influence than a payor who accounts for 35 percent of that group's dollars.

Taken in its totality, this wealth of very detailed payor mix market research will inform critical execution decisions about where your PSHP wants to compete (see Figures 3.4 and 3.5).

Concentration Dimensions	Some Implications of Low & High Concentration Levels
Payors	A low concentration of payors (commercial, Medicare and Medicaid) may mean that your delivery system is not at risk for retribution as it contracts with those same payors. However, it may mean that the market is crowded and it will not support another entrant. In a Medicaid environment, market share may be the result of regulation, while in a Medicare Advantage environment, the market may be immature.
	In addition to understanding the level of concentration you need to offer up a product for commercial, Medicare and Medicaid payors, you need to be acutely aware of other business issues that can change that concentration. For example, you might reevaluate offering a Medicare Advantage product as the age of Medicare-eligible consumers in your area becomes more heavily dominated by the younger Baby Boomers.
Employers and Their Employees	While employer-sponsored healthcare is shrinking, the group business on the commercial side is still the fastest way to aggregate a sufficient number of lives for a health plan. So if you are in a rural or semi-rural market, where a handful of employers provide a volume of lives and those lives typically get most of their care from providers in your plan, you could be ideally suited to work directly with those employers.
	If the commercial market is fragmented in terms of employers, it may mean you should think about selling your PSHP and its products on public and/or private exchanges.
	Aggregating lives in Medicaid differs by state and is obviously not employer-based. Similarly, the act of enrolling members into Medicare Advantage is a direct-to-consumer strategy unaffected by employer concentration. However, it potentially requires some of the same capabilities a PSHP uses to target consumers who buy healthcare insurance on exchanges.
Providers	The higher the provider concentration, or the greater the market share one healthcare organization has, the more control it has in terms of members and providers. Since many provider organizations are the only game in town, the key is to define your PSHP's primary service area in such a way that you ensure you have a broad enough number of both members and providers.
Interplay Between These Dimensions	On the commercial side, if payor, employer and provider concentrations are all high, your PSHP may be able to gain sufficient scale by working with a handful of employers. You also should protect your plan's providers from accepting poor rates from other insurance companies as retribution for taking some of their members away.

Source: Valence Health

Figure 3.4

Individual Market Share Snapshot

Source: Kaiser Health Facts

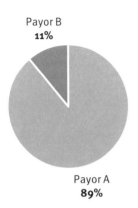

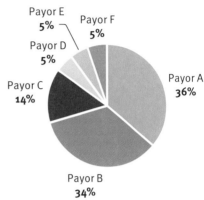

Certain areas of the United States contain a major payor that dominates the market. This payor can more easily influence providers through mechanisms like narrow networks.

In contrast, other parts of the country have multiple payors with modest market shares. This frequently empowers individual providers and healthcare organizations in contract negotiations.

Figure 3.5

Additionally, you also will need to determine how your new competitors will react to your health plan. As we mentioned in Chapter 1, "Why Should You Consider Starting a Provider-Sponsored Health Plan?," if one of your key PSHP's leadership team members currently receives 75 percent of his or her revenue from Blue Cross' commercial business, and Blue Cross refuses to renew that member's contract if it joins your PSHP, you may have to reevaluate.

In the end, as a new PSHP, you will be competing with other more experienced insurance companies. Using our bus analogy, your competitors will have established bus routes and dedicated or disgruntled riders (both members and healthcare providers). By creating tougher contract renewals, changing reimbursement rates or ending their contracts, established insurance companies can potentially try to take patients away from providers affiliated with your PSHP. As the new bus in town, you have to expect that your competitors may do just about anything to assure you are not successful. In this case, this is your chance to offer a better route to health or create value for affiliated providers in new and different ways.

Especially because we're provider-sponsored, we have an amazing opportunity before us. We have the opportunity to innovate. We've shortened the distance between the purchaser and the deliverer, and it's our obligation to figure out how to innovate in this space and make something better. That's what's exciting about this. It's the ultimate testing ground of what will come next."

– Stephen Nolte
CEO, Sutter Health Plus

Successful PSHPs constantly assess the different buses on the road and quickly identify which turns it wants and needs to take. Identifying where your health plan fits within the current competitive dynamic, and how much of the market share your health plan hopes to realistically capture, will go a long way in determining your execution strategy.

Assessing Provider Competition and Cooperation

In addition to competing with other health insurance companies, your organization will be competing with other health systems for market share in terms of patient volume. This brings up another very important question: Where do you rank against other providers in your market? Do the doctors, hospitals and other partners in your PSHP have:

- Higher, lower or similar quality scores?

- Equivalent accreditations?

- Higher, lower or similar geographic reach?

If you remember back to the Driscoll Children's Health Plan case study (discussed in Chapter 2, "How Today's PSHPs are Different"), Driscoll Children's Hospital is part of its PSHP and is 300 miles away from the next children's hospital. This makes it ideal for the health plan because the hospital commands the majority of market share for pediatric healthcare services, has strong brand recognition and enjoys a high level of consumer trust.

The higher the provider concentration or the greater the marker share one organization has, the more control it has in terms of patients and providers. Since many provider organizations are the only game in town, the key is to define your PSHP's primary service area in such a way that you ensure you have an adequate number of both patients and providers.

Keep in mind that many organizations, particularly those in large cities and perhaps even yours, have lower market shares due to high competition and a lack of services that set them apart. In these scenarios, organizations often partner with other health systems in the marketplace to increase their services, contracting abilities and geographic footprint. Forming alliances can certainly help differentiate PSHPs. As you think about why your PSHP should exist, carefully think about potential partners that fit into and philosophically support your vision and market penetration needs.

Identifying Your Available Consumer Base

Along with assessing patient volume, it is critical to review characteristics of the local patient population itself (see Figure 3.6). What are the demographic, economic and psychographic characteristics of your community and how will those characteristics change over time?

Key Consumer-Base Considerations for PSHPs

Source: Valence Health

Health Insurance Related Data Points	Consumer Preference
• On the commercial side, what is the percentage of fully insured versus self-insured employers? How big are the individual, small group and large markets in your area?	• What is the health club membership enrollment in your community?
• What is being offered on your state and federal exchange (if you have one) and what is successful?	• Which pharmacies fill the most prescriptions in your service area?
• What percentage of your population is Medicare-eligible?	• What are the most popular restaurants in your plan's primary geographic area?
• Of that group, how many are enrolled in Medicare Advantage plans and how many are not?	• What are the most heavily attended community events?
• What percentage are Medicaid-eligible?	• What transportation options are there for individuals who do not have access to a car? During what hours?
• How many are dual-eligible, or qualify for both Medicare and Medicaid benefits?	• What urgent care resources exist in your community?
	• Have other new businesses in your area conducted market research and could it relate to your potential consumer base?

Figure 3.6

Every population will have a different coverage mix and related healthcare preferences, and many will be very diverse. Remember, however, that your PSHP does not need to be all things to all people. This is where your value proposition comes in. The one thing you can do better than anyone else in the market is essential for determining who your target members should be.

Knowing which major lines of health insurance products your PSHP will sell also helps you determine how large your customer base needs to be profitable (see Figure 3.7). While there is always local flexibility, we have come to find that successful PSHPs insure a minimum number of lives.

Type of Insurance Product	Typical Total # of Members/ Lives Needed to Be Successful
Commercial	30,000 members
Medicare Advantage	10,000 members
Medicaid Managed Care	5,000 to 30,000 members depending on state-specific considerations, such as: • Total Medicaid-eligible population • Service area restrictions • Auto-assignment versus individual member choice

Source: Valence Health
Figure 3.7

Therefore, if there are only 3,000 Medicare-eligible individuals in your market, a Medicare Advantage (MA) product is not likely a good initial option for your PSHP. However, things change and a decision once made is just that, e.g., if a large successful assisted living chain decides to build a facility in your service area, your PSHP may opt to reconsider offering a MA product.

As you further define your consumer base, it also is valuable to note recent trends in consumer healthcare buying decisions. For example, the national push toward state and federal exchanges has revealed that while large employers typically prefer national insurance carriers, individual consumers tend to buy local trusted brands. The research coming back from employers that are using private exchanges also says that the price of different plan options is a huge factor.

As an example of knowing what consumers want, Land of Lincoln Health (see Figure 3.8), a health insurance Consumer-Operated-and-Oriented-Plan (CO-OP) based in Illinois, capitalized on a consumer reality. It found that public exchange consumers in the Chicago-metropolitan area trusted providers more than their payors, so the provider brand trumped the payor brand. Land of Lincoln Health leveraged this data to successfully enter a market that was dominated by one large commercial payor and by specifically marketing its provider-centric approach to health plan delivery. As a result, Land of Lincoln Health brought in more than 42,000 new members during the 2015 open enrollment timeframe for state and federal exchanges.

Land of Lincoln Health

Source: Valence Health

Land of Lincoln Health is the sole Consumer-Operated-and-Oriented-Plan (CO-OP) health insurance company in Illinois that was originally sponsored by a coalition of hospitals. This consumer-governed cooperative was sponsored by the Metropolitan Chicago Healthcare Council, a membership organization that assists more than 170 healthcare organizations with providing quality, accessible care to their communities in the Chicago area.

But what are CO-OPs, and how are they related to PSHPs? The CO-OP program was developed as part of the 2010 Affordable Care Act (ACA) and was made possible with low-interest federal loans. Designed to foster healthy competition in state marketplaces with more affordable, consumer-oriented health plan options, the CO-OPs are private, nonprofit health insurance companies.

Governed by the members, CO-OPs are fundamentally different from PSHPs in many ways, but they share many common goals. In particular, both health plan models strive to create forward-thinking, provider-friendly health plans that are responsive to the individual consumer and his or her needs.

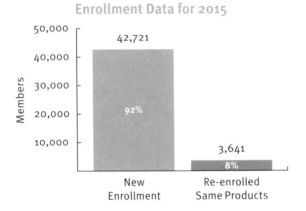

Figure 3.8

The Land of Lincoln Health is just one example that reinforces that in parts of the country with state and federal exchanges, it is very important for PSHPs to study what is happening to market share for exchange-supported individual and small group buyers. You will then want to compare this to what is happening in your commercial market or private employer-sponsored exchanges to note similarities and differences. These new options for buying health insurance are changing how the entire public makes health insurance selection decisions — including purchasing decisions about your plan. Learning what consumers look for on these exchanges and how to get your plan on applicable exchanges can help ensure your plan is a top contender (refer to Chapter 5, "Sales and Marketing," for more information on public and private insurance exchanges).

Since many public exchange members have lower income levels, they also may be more apt to move between Medicaid and public exchange coverage. Again, this heightens your need to understand what Medicaid is doing, especially in states that enacted both ACA-enabled public exchanges and Medicaid expansion.

To really know your customers, however, you need to know more than just their current coverage options. You need to get inside their heads and understand what really matters to your potential members. While there are increasing amounts of free and reasonably priced demographic, economic and psychographic data about smaller segments of the population, your PSHP will want to access different public and syndicated information that you may not have needed in your provider-only world.

You also have the opportunity to gather primary data by conducting focus groups or issuing surveys that ask current and potential consumers if they are happy with their current health benefits and healthcare outcomes. What features and coverage levels do they want to see in their health insurance plan? Which healthcare services do they use the most? What price are they willing to pay for a plan? In short, what is important to them? Finally, you need to understand the health status of your potential membership base (see Figure 3.9).

Examples of Useful Community Health Status Information for PSHPs

Source: Valence Health

- Incidence and prevalence statistics for certain conditions
- Public health data around things like immunization rates, pre-term births, teenage pregnancies, etc.
- Emergency room visits information per X number of members in a community
- Average facility census rates for all inpatient facilities in your service area

Figure 3.9

Identifying Regulatory Requirements

When analyzing your local healthcare landscape, you need to stay abreast of a whole new set of regulations that come with carrying a health insurance license. There will be a higher level of regulatory surveillance you will need to conduct. While some of these regulations are standard across the United States, many vary by state. If you are a PSHP that is targeting members from more than one state, you need to recognize that you will be increasing your work.

While we will discuss more about the regulatory realities of having a PSHP in Chapter 11, "Compliance," one notion that impacts your execution strategy is what we call regulatory PSHP "friendliness." In some states, there are laws and administrative rules that will make it more difficult for you to begin and compete on a level playing field. For example, some states might require that new health insurance companies hoping to operate in their state must have held a valid two-year insurance license in another state. In contrast, in some parts of the country, Medicaid may embrace PSHPs, but the Department of Insurance, which regulates commercial plans, may not.

Assessing Plan Readiness

After identifying your value proposition and completing your market analyses of your local health insurance ecosystem, it is time to take a reality check. Where is your organization now compared to where it needs to be when your plan goes live?

To find the answers to this question, we always counsel organizations to conduct a capabilities assessment or gap analysis. Oftentimes, this involves using base data from an experienced partner or advisor to identify gaps between your current operating abilities and recommended benchmarks.

> " Most providers are great at delivering outstanding patient care and service—that's what they do. However, they're not in the business of performing like a payor. Functions like sales, operations, claims, eligibility, member services—these support functions are not logical in a provider environment. Not only do we not speak the same language, but a provider isn't built to do those things. In fact, their entire culture and organization is built around many things that are just completely different than what insurance companies normally provide."
>
> **– Stephen Nolte**
> CEO, Sutter Health Plus

While every PSHP capabilities assessment conducted is different, the gaps tend to be in two critical areas: infrastructure and talent.

Infrastructure

Infrastructure is the body of your brand new PSHP "bus." For the bus to be the truly safe, efficient machine you wanted, the construction of each part must be exceptional.

Similarly, integrating a healthcare organization into the insurance industry requires a sound design to be successful (see Figure 3.10). This is primarily obvious in areas that must be developed from scratch.

Critical Health Plan Infrastructure Requirements

Source: Valence Health

Member Fulfillment
- ID card management
- Welcome packet fulfillment

Finance & Actuarial
- Broker commission management
- Employer group invoicing

Customer Support
- Call center operations
- Provider & member outreach
- Provider & member portals

Network Management
- Network development
- Negotiations
- Provider credentialing & relations

Eligibility & Capitation
- Financial management & budgeting
- Risk modeling
- Financial statistical reporting
- Experience rebates

Broker Management
- X12 834 eligibility data
- Reconciliation
- Premium receipt & validation

Reporting
- Operational
- OB 837
- Medical
- Analytical

Care Management
- Utilization management, case management, disease management and population health
- Social service outreach
- Quality improvement & clinical initiative support
- Reports, analytics & certification support: HEDIS, etc.
- Patient engagement
- 24/7 RN line

Claims Management
- Claim payment & explanation of benefits/explanation of payment production
- Coordination with special investigations unit
- Fee schedule management
- Encounter data capture

Figure 3.10

For example, healthcare organizations typically do not have a customer service department that addresses providers' and members' needs and questions. Nor do providers have actuarial departments or the information technology resources to pay claims, automate parts of case and disease management information, and integrate health plan data back into electronic medical records. As a stand-alone provider, you simply did not need the infrastructure that is required by a health plan.

For those functions that exist within your current provider organization — like sales and marketing, financial management and network management — you will have to make another set of executional strategy decisions. Do you divide current resources into two separate teams or share resources among your health system and PSHP respectively?

While you may have access to functions like utilization management, case management and compliance from your provider organization, you will have to understand the degree of investment needed to ensure current departments can meet health insurance compliance standards and operating benchmarks. This raises questions like:

- Do we increase the number of proactive disease, case management and care coordination programs we offer?

- Can current case mangers handle the new workloads?

- How will we calculate return on investment (ROI) for the health system and the health plan?

- As a health plan, can we accept full responsibility for identifying systemic problems among our providers that are driving up costs and put programs in place to eliminate or reduce them?

Not surprisingly, when we have completed PSHP capability gap assessment projects, we often find huge gaps. While these gaps are often daunting, your comprehensive execution strategy will help determine the most effective and practical solutions for closing them. The important thing to know now is just how far your PSHP will need to go to successfully meet the standards and benchmarks needed to keep your PSHP bus running with a full tank of gas.

Talent

If infrastructure is the body of your bus, talent is the oil that keeps the engine running smoothly. Even though your current staff may be amazing, their strengths may or may not help you succeed as a PSHP. As we have worked with provider organizations on every kind of risk-arrangement imaginable, we have seen time and time again that as providers accept greater financial risk for patients and populations, they need front-line leaders with both insurance and clinical experience to succeed. As a result, organizations like Valence Health often provide interim executives and/or mentor other professionals to help the talent pool at the PSHP prepare for different roles. As a result, the PSHP bus gets better mileage.

Therefore, to run a successful health plan, you need executives who have expertise in:

- Actuarial and financial disciplines and how to price plans to meet insurance commissioner reporting requirements and identify capital inadequacies

- Marketing and sales, and are familiar with regulations surrounding what information can and cannot be used in health plan selection advertising and communications

In short, you likely will need additional staff as well as staff with different expertise. A comprehensive talent assessment will help you determine just how many and what kind of professionals you will need to have on your bus' maintenance team.

> ### Expert Insight
>
> *"There are successful PSHPs that choose to build separate and discrete functions from those that exist in the provider's non-health plan organization. Human resources (HR) is a perfect example. We have counseled some of our clients to hire their own PSHP HR director right away and before many of the senior management positions are filled. This creates two distinct advantages. First, it frees up the PSHP's leadership, allowing them to focus on other business issues that are critical in the initial stages of a plan's development. Second, it allows the HR professional to outline the distinct skills and attributes that will be needed when hiring team members for the plan's start-up phase."*
>
> **– Karen Janousek**
> President, Health Plan Services, Valence Health

Getting to the Starting Line

The good news is that your transition to a PSHP can be made at whatever speed you like. You can crawl, walk or run as you seek to operationalize your health plan (see Figures 3.11 and 3.12).

When starting a PSHP, some groups choose to start small and limit their scope of business. For example, some PSHPs start by piloting a Medicare Advantage product, which may be somewhat easier to market since it is sold directly to individuals. Over time, you can then decide if you want to expand your consumer base to encompass more segments of the population or other lines of business. By slowly increasing your membership, you can be more conscious of building products or offerings that are within the bounds of your existing infrastructure, talent and financial resources.

Alternatively, other PSHPs put their gas pedals fully to the metal. There are very successful PSHPs and CO-OPs that launched with diverse product offerings and purposefully wanted to get as many members as quickly as possible. Their execution strategy is more revolutionary than evolutionary, and takes advantage of business opportunities that sometimes come with scale.

Risk Level & Required Provider Capabilities for Value-Based Care

Source: Valence Health & McClellan, et al., "A National Strategy to Put Accountable Care into Practice" Health Affairs, May 2010

	LEVEL ONE: CIN/Pay for Performance	**LEVEL TWO:** Shared Savings Model	**LEVEL THREE:** Risk Share, Bundled Payments	**LEVEL FOUR:** Capitation, up to Full Risk	**LEVEL FIVE:** Capitation including Claims Payment	**LEVEL SIX:** Provider as the Health Plan
	Crawl		**Walk**		**Run**	
Metrics and Provider Payment Models	• Legal entity with basic health IT and performance reporting capabilities • Core "starter set" of quality, efficiency and patient-experience measures	• Strong infrastructure (advanced health IT, care coordination staff) • Shared savings for meeting quality and spending targets; no downside risk	• Strong infrastructure (advanced health IT, care coordination staff) • Making transition to advanced measure emphasizing health outcomes, function status and reductions in health risk • Larger shared savings balanced by accountability for costs exceeding targets	• Advanced infrastructure, full range of services, reserve requirements • Stronger/more performance targets and reporting requirements • Risk-adjusted partial capitation payments with quality bonuses	• Advanced infrastructure, full range of services, reserve requirements • Stronger/more performance targets and reporting requirements • Capitation with quality bonuses; adjudicating claims and making payments to providers	• Advanced infrastructure, full range of services, reserve requirements • Full health plan functionality • Full health plan functionality

Figure 3.11

Responsibility Matrix for Delivering Key Aspects of Value-Based Care

Legend:
- ◑ Health Plan
- ● Shared
- ◐ Provider/Accountable Care Organization
- ○ Not Applicable
- ⊘ Capabilities that can be provided by Valence Health

		Crawl	Walk		Run		
		LEVEL ONE: CIN/Pay for Performance	LEVEL TWO: Shared Savings Model	LEVEL THREE: Risk Share, Bundled Payments	LEVEL FOUR: Capitation, up to Full Risk	LEVEL FIVE: Capitation including Claims Payment	LEVEL SIX: Provider as the Health Plan
Marketing & Sales							
⊘	Underwriting	◑	◑	◑	◑	◑	◐
⊘	Premium billing & accounting	◑	◑	◑	◑	◑	◐
⊘	Benefit plan design/plan documents	◑	◑	◑	◑	◑	◐
	Group sales	◑	◑	◑	◑	◑	◐
	Individual sales	◑	◑	◑	◑	◑	◐
Legal & Regulatory							
⊘	Rate filings	◑	◑	◑	◑	◑	◐
⊘	Licensure	◑	◑	◑	◑	◑	◐
⊘	State reporting	◑	◑	◑	◑	◑	◐
⊘	Provider regulatory process (TBD)	◐	◐	◐	◐	◐	◐
Risk & Financial Management							
⊘	Finance & accounting	◑	◑	●	●	●	◐
⊘	IBNR (Incurred But Not Reported)	◑	◑	●	●	●	◐
⊘	Actuarial analysis	◑	◑	●	●	●	◐
	Reserves	◑	◑	◑	●	●	◐
	Reinsurance	◑	◑	●	●	●	◐
⊘	Rate development	◑	◑	◑	◑	◑	◐
Claims							
⊘	Claims receipt & processing	◑	◑	◑	◑	◐	◐
⊘	Benefit determination	◑	◑	◑	◑	◐	◐
⊘	Claims adjudication & payment	◑	◑	◑	◑	◐	◐
⊘	Claim audits	◑	◑	◑	◑	◐	◐
⊘	COB/subrogation	◑	◑	◑	◑	◐	◐
Shared Savings/Bonus Cap Payment							
	Attribute member to the ACO	◑	◑	◑	◑	◑	◑
	Reconcile & pay bonus to ACO	◑	◑	◑	◑	◑	◑
	Bundled payments to ACO	○	○	◑	○	○	○
⊘	Capitation to ACO	○	○	○	◑	◑	○
⊘	Distribution within ACO	◐	◐	◐	◐	◐	◐

Figure 3.12

In full transparency, there are advantages and disadvantages associated with both approaches. For example, expensive or high-dollar claims may be more difficult for small plans to manage because they collect less premium revenue. For PSHPs that make their transition at 55 miles per hour, the ability to have a large customer service staff that can handle multiple lines of business may prove to be very difficult and expensive. While we have seen both approaches work and fail, be sure that your organization wrestles with and fully owns the approach.

Closing Your Operational Gaps

Given the strengths and weaknesses that you identify, your PSHP will need to know how it will access the necessary infrastructure, functionality and required talent to reach and hopefully exceed industry-accepted benchmarks (see Figure 3.13). While there is no perfect bus blueprint, there are several best practices that organizations can use when deciding to build, buy or partner/outsource various operations and functions (see Figure 3.14 for the pros and cons of each choice).

Options for Adding New PSHP Operating Capabilities

Source: Valence Health

When a provider decides to launch its own health plan, the organization is immersed in the typically unfamiliar waters of insurance and risk management. There are four basic ways to add these new insurance and risk management capabilities:

- **Build**—Working from the ground up, providers can develop these capabilities internally, hiring personnel and implementing the necessary technologies
- **Buy**—The provider organization can acquire the assets and personnel of an existing health plan
- **Partner**—The provider organization can partner with an existing plan, leveraging that organization's technology, people and infrastructure
- **Outsource**—In this model, the provider organization handles some of the payor responsibilities while outsourcing other functions that remain under the provider's brand and guidance

Figure 3.13

As your PSHP continues to grow, your operations and functional departments should be regularly reevaluated. What may have made sense to do with two employees when you had less than 2,000 members may not make sense when you have more than 12,000 members. Whether just beginning your PSHP or making updates, a build, buy or partner/outsource analyses is always a critical part of your ongoing comprehensive execution strategy.

Advantages and Disadvantages with Different Execution Strategy Options

Source: Valence Health

Model	Pros	Cons
Build	• Control • Specificity of design	• $10–$20 million in start-up costs, plus risk-based capital • Execution risk due to lack of experience
Buy	• Immediate capability • Experienced operators	• Scarce supply of assets to buy • Very expensive costs between $500–$1,000 per covered life
Partner	• Immediate capability • Experienced operators	• Scarce supply of partners • Possible misalignment of incentives • Lack of control
Outsource	• Immediate capability • Experienced operators • Can custom-design relationships	• Few experienced vendors • Requires relationship management

Figure 3.14

#1: Building PSHP Operations to Match Your Strengths

There are certain tasks that your PSHP will likely want to build internally. Although this can be a lengthy and expensive process, this gives your organization full control to design and staff those functional areas. When organizations do build their own, you have the opportunity to reinforce your providers' strengths.

For example, critically examine your value proposition and your brand recognition. What differentiates your organization from all of your peers? These key components — these strengths — are core to your organization's identity and should probably be built in-house.

Case Study:
Owning What is Unique to You

"As we created a health plan, we knew right away that we wanted to own the way we communicated with members and to create a different member experience. We spent a lot of time thinking through health insurance literacy. To get to where we wanted to be, we partnered with experts from Northwestern University and Emory University to help us adopt a health literacy lens in creating every one of our materials. Our members' experiences, our voice and our communication with both our stakeholders and our members — that is a space we needed to own."

– Jason Montrie
President, Land of Lincoln Health

Due to the highly variable nature of the insurance industry and regulatory agencies' increased scrutiny surrounding all health plans' processes, many PSHPs build their own compliance and regulatory reporting functions. For example, Medicare Advantage plans work extensively with Centers for Medicare & Medicaid Services (CMS). Therefore, many PSHPs also feel their own compliance staff can more effectively receive guidance from regulatory agencies regarding rules and requirements by communicating directly with them as opposed to going through a third party administrator (TPA).

Compliance staff also needs a deep understanding of your organization and its products. Your plan's processes will be evaluated and updated continuously to ensure they comply with current and new regulations. As told in the following case study, many organizations, like Dean Health Plan, therefore prefer to have in-house compliance staff (for more information, refer to Chapter 11, "Compliance").

Case Study:
Maintaining Compliance with New Regulations

"After the ACA was implemented, it became clear that the compliance department at Dean Health Plan needed additional help to maintain compliance. There were too many regulations being released and many of the topics were areas that our compliance professionals knew little about. For example, they received new technology specifications for electronic transactions between CMS and our health plan, but we had no idea how to modify the current technology to meet those specifications.

To improve the process, we identified a compliance professional in each functional area and registered that person to receive the regulators' emails and webinar training notices. If a new information technology (IT) regulation came out, then just the professional in that functional area would discuss with the compliance leadership team how the new regulation would impact the plan without involving other compliance staff.

This structure is still in place today, and all the functional areas gather for quarterly or monthly meetings to talk about potential audits, what they have learned in conferences and other relevant topics. It allows us to function efficiently, while still staying connected in the organization."

– Christine Senty
Former General Counsel, Dean Health Plan

#2: Outsourcing Your Weaknesses

In the end, it is much better to know your weaknesses than to be surprised by them. It also is much easier to address operational weaknesses if they are commodity-like parts for your PSHP's "bus" and then find a trusted partner to collaborate with.

The truth is, an outside partner, often referred to as a TPA, will have the trained staff and core technology to help you to address your weakness. If your organization cannot afford to miss the mark, many PSHPs choose to outsource various back-office functions and operational necessities of the health insurance industry, like claims processing (see Figure 3.15). The high cost and experience required to properly build, buy or partner/outsource a claims processing platform deters many PSHPs, particularly because the complexity of these platforms increases with the number of enrollees in any health plan. This area also demands a team of knowledgeable staff with skills that are tailored to paying claims according to your PSHP's contracts rules and timeframes (for more information on claims processing, refer to Chapter 9, "Claims Administration and Management").

Commonly Outsourced PSHP Functions	Additional Discussion
• Claims Processing	Chapter 9, "Claims Administration and Management"
• Customer Service	Chapter 8, "Customer Service"
• Broker Management	Chapter 5, "Sales and Marketing"
• Disease Management	Chapter 7, "Medical Management"
• Actuarial and Analytic Services	Chapter 10, "Actuarial Considerations and Financial Management"

Source: Valence Health
Figure 3.15

Clearly the biggest advantages of working with a partner is that it saves you time and lets you allocate your own resources to other issues. With the right partner, your PSHP's leadership team can focus on other aspects of the health plan, while knowing critical jobs are getting done. With a great partner, there is ongoing teaching and mentoring so that business responsibilities can be seamlessly passed back and forth as demands ebb and flow.

#3: Ensuring Maximum Return on Your Build, Buy or Partnership/Outsourcing Decisions

Ultimately, your decision to build, buy or partner/outsource various PSHP functions will depend on your ROI analyses. From our 20 years of experience, it is impractical to think you can build everything in-house, but we also have seen that internal operations can be as effective as many outsourced pieces. The critical question is, at what expense? What trade-offs are you making to gain competitive parity or advantages?

Most likely, the complexity of each PSHP function as compared to the costs of the function will heavily influence your choices. Operating elements for some PSHP products are relatively simple and do not require large investments. For example, take the accounting process for some Medicaid managed care products. The premiums and eligibility files are provided to you by a state agency and a cash transfer goes into your bank account.

However, more complex processes, like premium billing members who have commercial plans, cannot be implemented without a major investment. (For more information on accounting, refer to Chapter 10, "Actuarial Considerations and Financial Management." For more information on premium billing, refer to Chapter 9, "Claims Administration and Management").

Always Keep Your Eyes on the Road

While your PSHP might start out small, the number and types of "bus" riders you manage will change over time due to fluctuating enrollment numbers and demographics. This means that the functional components you ultimately decide to build, buy or partner/outsource need to be expandable and flexible. Those same principles hold true for your staff and infrastructure. A benefit to partnering with another company is that your organization can collaborate to create a long-term project plan. This allows you to visualize how your PSHP and partnerships will evolve as your plan changes.

For example, while it may be initially more judicious to outsource utilization management (UM) and case management (CM) services, some PSHPs eventually move some or all of these areas in-house once they have reached 40,000 to 50,000 lives/members (for more information on UM and CM, refer to Chapter 7, "Medical Management"). For these very reasons, Valence Health has adapted its UM and CM support models to provide a range of UM or CM services, whether that involves providing additional staff resources to clients (be they nurses or community health workers) or provision of case management technology that the PSHP's staff will use. We believe that this type of a modular PSHP execution strategy gives our clients time to flexibly deploy resources, while knowing they have operational spare tires or professional back-up when needed.

Maintaining Accountability

Hopefully, the best practices and the functionally specific roles discussed in this part of Chapter 3 will give your plan's leaders a sense for how they might tackle their own build, buy or partner/outsource decisions. However, regardless of what options you select, you will need processes and metrics in place to hold both internal and external staff responsible for meeting agreed-upon business objectives.

As we always tell our clients, the outsourced components of your PSHP are not any less your own. You are still responsible for their successes and their failures. To address this, some organizations have vendor relationship managers to ensure their PSHP has control of their partnerships. This manager monitors and challenges the performance of a plan's partners to protect the organization's interests. Through hands-on, interactive discussions, the vendor relationship manager reviews current processes and discusses strategic enhancements to continuously improve performance.

Best practice vendor relationship managers also get out of the office to assist with training their partners. Consider the opportunities created when customer service representatives (CSRs) work side by side with some of your plan's leadership team. Since your health plan and your geographic area are unique, it often is helpful to provide terminology and knowledge that will enable CSRs to become local market experts. In turn, CSRs can share their learnings with the PSHP's executives. For example, have they found a particularly effective way to explain your plan's benefits that you can use in other sales and marketing activities?

For every function you perform, your PSHP also will need an organization and governance structure that ensures accountability. Regardless of your decision to combine or separate functions, you need to encourage cross-pollination, pursue innovations and prevent conflicts of interest that come from running two connected, but in some cases, competing businesses.

 I'm mindful of the fact there has to be a line in the sand between a payor and a provider organization. At Sutter Health Plus, we were able to share several best practices and proven processes already in place in the provider side of the organization. But we couldn't homogenize everything. There's a delicate balance to strike between the obligations of a payor and that of a provider. A payor organization can't be compromised by becoming too much like the provider. On the other hand, the provider has to recognize that it can't be the health plan. Each organization has strengths—and weaknesses—it needs to recognize to be successful."

– Stephen Nolte
CEO, Sutter Health Plus

In that vein, many PSHPs find it to be a good business sense to have two separate UM and financial management functions — one for the health plan and the other for its hospitals — because the staff performing these jobs has very different objectives. For example, in UM, when a PSHP has two different departments, you can separate the nurses who request authorizations from the nurses who approve or deny them.

> **Expert Insight**
>
> *"If you create a PSHP, you need to have a completely separate team managing the health plan. So you are going to have your hospital business and all of the employees that manage that business in one silo, and you are going to have a health plan team in another silo. There will be multiple touch points between the two groups, but you should never have the hospital financial folks playing a role in the health plan's finances. They are two different animals with very different skill sets. The trick is to create a forum to ensure that cross-learning and education occurs. You have to be vigilant in making sure silos are never counterproductive."*
>
> **– Steve Tutewohl**
> Strategic Accounts Officer, Valence Health

Do not forget, however, that as a PSHP, you have the freedom to design organizational rules that will make these interactions more productive than they might be in other health insurance organizations.

For example, a PSHP can bring together a cross-section of UM nurses to establish specific criteria for determining if a certain procedure is medically necessity. Even though the PSHP's nurses may have to deny some of the hospital nurses' requests, the creation of a shared set of rules may result in less animosity and create more impactful and effective guidelines (for more information on financial management, refer to Chapter 7, "Medical Management" and Chapter 10, "Actuarial Considerations and Financial Management").

Likewise, PSHPs must perform internal audits to ensure their current processes are satisfying established compliance requirements and quality benchmarks. These audits can be performed by in-house or external auditors. While the supervisors, managers and directors of a PSHP's operational departments may be good at auditing their own staff members, they often have difficulty identifying the problems and necessary changes in departmental processes because they have written them themselves. For this reason, many PSHPs value the objective audit results from independent auditors (for more information on internal audits, refer to Chapter 11, "Compliance").

Considering Your Finances

Now that you have a working value proposition and a thoughtful and comprehensive execution strategy to run your PSHP, you need to make sure you have enough gas in the tank to get you where you need to go (see Figure 3.16). In other words, you need to examine your total cost and revenue structure by evaluating your:

- One-time and ongoing costs infrastructure

- Expected revenues

- Other sources of capital

- Expected pay-back requirements and expectations

Illustrative

Start-Up Costs*	
Implementation Costs	$500,00
Staff (comp, facility)	$4,500,000
Legal/Consulting	$1,000,000
Other	$500,000
Total	$6,500,000
Risk-Based Capital	$15,300,000
Total Initial Required Capital	$21,800,000

Ongoing Financials*	PMPM	Annual
Total Premium	$150.00	$1,80,000,000
Medical Costs	$132.08	$158,500,000
Operations	$4.17	$5,000,000
Admin/Medical Management	$8.50	$10,200,00
Premium Tax	$3.00	$3,600,00
Profit	$2.25	$2,700,00
Payback Period	2.4 Years	
*Assumes 100,000 members		

Source: Valence Health
Figure 3.16

You need to be as accurate as possible when answering cost-related questions because it will directly impact what price you can charge certain payors, specifically employers and consumers. In Medicare and Medicaid, while your plan price or per-member per-month (PMPM) reimbursement will be determined by a set of regulations, you still need to understand all aspects of that pricing. Bottom line: any price for any product will impact how much revenue your plan can bring in. This, in turn, determines what your PSHP can pay its hospitals and physicians.

You also need to determine your risk-based capital requirements as well as your reserves. Successful PSHPs also consider their products and line-of-business pricing structure when creating reserves. For example, if you know that your pricing is more aggressive, then you will want more reserves on-hand to cover potential losses.

As your organization makes these decisions, you may realize that you need additional capital to finance your PSHP. If so, then you are in good company. Probably 80 percent to 90 percent of PSHPs, if not more, are financially backed by one or more hospitals. If your PSHP is affiliated with a hospital or health system, odds are this partner may invest a portion of its money into the health plan. This affiliation can even help reduce your capital requirements and benefit your bottom line, depending on how your contract is written.

Some PSHPs form a contract between the health plan and hospital that guarantees the hospital will become full owners of the health plan in the event of a default. This type of agreement allows the health plan to classify certain requirements and expenses differently when reporting them to the state.

Other less-frequent means of attaining capital include approaching a payor or another partner, like a bank or a private equity firm, for help. Lastly, providers who are offering a Medicaid product also can approach their state government and request assistance so they can help make the market more competitive.

If your total cost structure and the prospect of borrowing large sums of capital seem daunting, bear in mind that your PSHP is an investment. You will need to put in money upfront, but by year three, many successful PSHPs see a positive ROI. Many plans opt to think and spend like a startup to help endure the variability and unpredictability that comes with any new business. No matter what the approach, successful plans ultimately know if they can live with any costs and revenue imbalance and for how long.

Lastly, you will need to decide what to do with your PSHP's profits. This includes determining how you will invest or spend the profits/revenues and what percentage will be given to network providers. At Valence Health, we believe that your organization's mission and motivation for becoming a PSHP should drive this decision (for more information on financial management, refer to Chapter 10, "Actuarial Considerations and Financial Management").

Evaluating Progress and Making Adjustments to Your Bus Route

In addition to the required reporting you will have to undertake as a PSHP, patients, employers, physicians and elected officials are demanding more accountability for healthcare costs and quality. Therefore, once you have set your comprehensive execution strategy, you will need to be vigilant about tracking and reporting on your performance (see Figure 3.17).

Sample PSHP Performance Report

Source: Valence Health

Financial and Operational Snapshot (does not include incurred but not reported (IBNR))				
	Reported Year to Date	Budget Year to Date	Prior Year to Date	Prior Year Total	Calendar Year Projected Total
Covered Lives	18,572	18,000	16,899	18,629	20,473
Member Months	109,784	108,000	98,358	206,871	219,568
Premium Revenue	$38,161,348	$36,819,438	$33,688,235	$72,013,894	$76,322,696
Other Income	$457,753	$566,748	$539,078	$1,078,156	$915,506
Total Revenue	$38,619,101	$37,386,186	$34,227,313	$73,092,050	$77,238,202
Medical & Drug Expenses	$32,170,475	$30,858,480	$26,718,682	$25,173,971	$64,340,950
Admin & Other Expenses	$6,293,961	$5,980,062	$6,366,117	$12,732,234	$12,587,922
Total Expenses	$38,464,436	$36,838,542	$33,084,799	$37,906,025	$76,928,872
Net Income Before Taxes	$154,665	$547,644	$1,142,514	$35,186,025	$309,330
Generally Accepted Accounting Principle Adjustments & Taxes	$18,013	-$191,676	-$390,297	$0	$36,026
Reported Net Income	$172,678	$355,968	$752,217	$35,186,025	$345,356

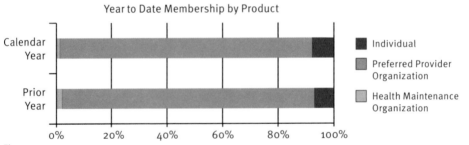

Year to Date Membership by Product

- Individual
- Preferred Provider Organization
- Health Maintenance Organization

Figure 3.17

While "Actuarial Considerations and Financial Management" and "Compliance" are explored in greater detail in Chapters 10 and 11 respectively, PSHPs typically need to give added attention to two specific elements. First, if your governing body is made up of various community stakeholders who do not have health insurance backgrounds, you will need to devote time to educating them to ensure there is a level playing field when sharing information about and interpreting the results of your PSHP's performance.

Second, if you go back to your PSHP's value proposition, your broader management team also will need to decide how it will share metrics related specifically to that value proposition among internal and external stakeholders. Will you need unique measures to capture the value of your local brand or the ability to more appropriately keep members in-network?

Since PSHPs should be in greater direct touch with their members, you will have to decide how to most immediately and fairly report on health outcomes and cost trends. As innovators, PSHPs have the rare opportunity to push themselves beyond standard evaluation metrics and find unique approaches to performance monitoring and reporting that make a difference for the patients, providers and payors they represent.

Evolving Your PSHP to Address Changing Times: Growing Alliant Health Plans

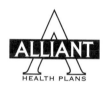

Alliant Health Plans (Alliant) has been operating as a nonprofit provider-sponsored healthcare corporation in northwest Georgia since 1998. Alliant insures approximately 30,000 commercial lives; equally comprised of employees and individual health plan purchasers. The payor is jointly owned by Hamilton Health Care System and Physicians Health Services (PHS) in Dalton, Ga., a small town that's earned the nickname "carpet capital of the world" due to the large volume of carpet and related businesses located there.

Hamilton Medical Center, the system's flagship hospital, is a longstanding and well-respected beacon in the community that has been recognized many times over for its clinical excellence, most recently with the 2015 Medical Excellence Award. The 282-bed medical center is the largest hospital in the surrounding counties. Its rich history and reputation for providing a high quality of care has earned Hamilton unwavering trust in the tight-knit community it serves.

PHS is a regional Independent Practice Association (IPA) consisting of approximately 195 doctors representing multiple specialties. It is currently the area's largest IPA.

Hamilton Health and PHS's history with Alliant is storied. In the mid-1990s, Hamilton was one of several health systems that had joint ownership of the health plan. Cognizant of its members' allegiance and recognizing the opportunity for continued market opportunity created by providing low-cost, high-value health insurance products, Hamilton joined with PHS in 1998 and took 50/50 ownership of Alliant. The buyout was a strategic move to further both owners' geographic reach, establish greater autonomy around how care is delivered and managed, provide small employers with more insurance options, and gain increased leverage and negotiating power in conversations with other regional and national health plans.

> ### Alliant Leverages Valence Health's Full Suite of TPA Managed Services Including:
>
> - Population technology solutions including Valence Health vElect©, Valence Health vCare© and Valence Health vQuest© applications
> - Analytics and reporting support
> - Data management
> - Member and provider enrollment and eligibility support
> - Finance and actuarial support
>
> - Full claims administration and management
> - Medical and broker management
> - Member fulfillment
> - Member and provider customer service
> - Member, employer, broker and provider portal provisions
> - Advisory/consulting services

Source: Alliant Health Plans
Figure 3.18

The partnership between Alliant and Valence Health began in 2002 when Alliant reevaluated its comprehensive execution strategy. Having decided to partner with an integrated end-to-end value-based care provider, Alliant turned to Valence Health to initially help the plan improve select back-office operations. Over the past decade, the two organizations have come to work hand-in-hand, with Valence Health taking on a full range of the plan's TPA responsibilities (see Figure 3.18).

"In addition to maintaining our core managed services, we have greater insight into what has and hasn't been done well in similar scenarios in other markets, and an ability to make sense of our own data," said Mark Mixer, Chief Operating Officer of Alliant.

At that point, Alliant had become a well-respected health insurance option for Northwest, Georgia residents. Over the past few years, Alliant saw an opportunity to further strengthen its network. When the ACA was signed into law in 2010 and the Federally Facilitated Marketplace (FFM) Exchanges were created, the plan saw a prime opportunity to again maintain and grow its membership.

FFM enrollment among Alliant members rose 154 percent between 2014 and 2015. Part of its FFM performance success can be attributed to Alliant qualifying as a National Committee for Quality Assurance (NCQA) accredited health plan, and developing a wrap network to expand its geographic reach. Alliant also began using integrated business intelligence tools and Valence Health technology to specifically support its medical spending analysis and utilization trends to refine its product offerings in 2015.

Alliant's success is a testament to the importance of providing best-in-class core payor services that are deeply attuned to a local community's needs and wants (see Figure 3.19). While Hamilton Medical Center and PHS aren't the only option for residents in nearby communities, these two organizations are viewed as the go-to area hospital and physicians group, both for convenience, as well as for the quality services they provide.

 Given its forward-looking strategic approach to serving its community, Alliant has experienced nearly 10 straight years of profitability and steady growth."

– Mark Mixer
Chief Operating Officer, Alliant Health Plans

There are other success factors at play, too. Hamilton and PHS have excelled at collaborating for the greater good of the health plan, and Alliant, in turn, has implemented an advanced shared-savings program with its IPA physicians and employed doctors. Each party is acutely aware of the role it plays in the overall partnership, constantly working to balance the needs of Alliant's institutional and individual healthcare provider partners.

Alliant Health Plans – A Part of the Community

Source: Alliant Health Plans

In addition to providing health plan services, Alliant has woven itself into the community fabric of Northwest, Ga. by:
• Providing college scholarships to local high school students
• Sponsoring local sporting competitions supporting charity
• Hosting community health fairs
• Assuring community members sit on plan's board

Figure 3.19

Today, the health plan, the hospital and the IPA — view their partnership as a strategic investment to better serve their constituents. According to Mark Mixer, "It's impossible to embark on true population health management without an element of risk, and our new approach to services and data intelligence has enabled us to not only manage a population, but to identify that population. We've successfully navigated this new model of care to the benefit of our patients."

Alliant also reflects a core element of many other successful provider-owned strategies: the need to begin with an intense focus and in-depth understanding of one's existing market, then form strategic partnerships with like-minded organizations to reach new constituencies. Alliant's successes to date have encouraged the plan's leadership to once again consider additional strategic expansion, which will enable Alliant to continually provide the best value to providers, employers and members for their premium dollars. ⊘

Tracking Key Health Plan Execution Strategy Metrics

Performing regular data analysis can help your PSHP maximize its return on investment and identify both early warning signs of trouble and indicators of success. By tracking key inputs and outputs, you can continually enhance your health plan so it retains members, remains financially stable and earns high patient satisfaction scores. Below are key execution strategy metrics that should be measured continuously:

- Overall payor competition analysis, including other payors' revenue, medical and administrative costs and average number of members by line of business
- Your plan's projected market share
- Your plan's patient volume
- Member coverage mix

- Time and cost requirements for creating each needed department/function
- ROI for creating each department/ function
- Total cost structure and plan pricing
- Governmental impact on your cost structure

Industry Terminology Related to Determining Your PSHP's Comprehensive Execution Strategy

Customer Service Representative Employee responsible for maintaining goodwill between a business organization and its customers by answering questions, solving problems and providing advice or assistance in utilizing the goods or services of the organization.

Source: AllBusiness.com

Electronic Medical Record A real-time patient health record with access to evidence-based decision support tools that can be used to aid clinicians in decision making. The EMR can automate and streamline a clinician's workflow, ensuring that all clinical information is communicated. It can also prevent delays in response that result in gaps in care. The EMR can also support the collection of data for uses other than clinical care, such as billing, quality management, outcome reporting and public health disease surveillance and reporting. Synonymous with Electronic Health Record or EHR.

Source: Office of the National Coordinator for Health IT

High-Dollar Claims Expensive health services such as organ transplants or long-term cancer treatments.

Source: HHC Insurance Holdings, Inc.

Independent Practice Association (IPA) A legal entity organized and directed by physicians in private practice to negotiate contracts with insurance companies on their behalf. Participating physicians are usually paid on a capitated or modified fee-for-service basis and may also continue to care for patients not covered by the insurers with whom the IPA contracts. Perhaps the most significant function of an IPA is to exert influence on behalf of its members to counterbalance the leverage of healthcare insurers. Synonymous with Independent Physicians Association.

Source: RiverCity Medical Group

Medicaid Expansion The Affordable Care Act provides states with additional federal funding to expand their Medicaid programs to cover adults under 65 with income up to 133% of the federal poverty level. Children (18 and under) are eligible up to that income level or higher in all states. This means that in states that have expanded Medicaid, free or low-cost health coverage is available to people with incomes below a certain level regardless of disability, family status, financial resources and other factors that are usually taken into account in Medicaid eligibility decisions.

Source: Healthcare.gov

National Association of Insurance Commissioners (NAIC) The U.S. standard-setting and regulatory support organization created and governed by the chief insurance regulators from the 50 states, the District of Columbia and five U.S. territories. Through the NAIC, state insurance regulators establish standards and best practices, conduct peer review and coordinate their regulatory oversight.

Source: NAIC

Open Enrollment A period of time, usually but not always occurring once per year, when employees of companies and organizations may make changes to their elected fringe benefit options, such as health insurance. The term also applies to the annual period during which individuals may buy individual health insurance plans through the online, state-based health insurance exchanges established by the Patient Protection and Affordable Care Act.

Source: Wikipedia.org

Reserves The money a company or individual keeps on-hand to meet its short-term and emergency funding needs.

Source: Investopedia.com

Return on Investment (ROI) A performance measure used to evaluate the efficiency of an investment or to compare the efficiency of a number of different investments.

Source: Investopedia.com

Risk-Based Capital (RBC)   In health insurance, RBC rules establish the minimum required liquid assets or cash reserves that health plans must have on-hand. Risk-based capital requirements exist to protect the firms, their investors and customers and the economy as a whole. Placement of risk-based capital requirements ensure that each financial institution has enough capital to sustain operating losses, while maintaining a safe and efficient market.

Source: Investopedia.com/terms

Third-Party Administrator (TPA)   A person or organization that processes claims and performs other administrative services in accordance with a service contract, usually in the field of employee benefits. More specifically, a TPA is neither the insurer (provider) nor the insured (employees or plan participants), but handles the administration of the plan including processing, adjudication, and negotiation of claims, recordkeeping and maintenance of the plan.

Source: MyCafeteriaPlan.com

Wrap Network   Wrap networks provide access to in-network providers, hospitals and ancillary services throughout the nation, providing a broad network for when your members are out of area and require medical care. Most PSHPs form a single contract with a national preferred provider organization (PPO) network to form a wrap network. Plan members can identify the wrap network from their ID card and hopefully access the closest in-network provider.

Source: Valence Health

Chapter Four
Plan Design

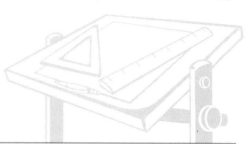

One of the most critical things your provider-sponsored health plan (PSHP) team will do is to design your product offerings or the types of health plans you will offer. In other words, it is time to build a better bus (see Figure 4.1). These plans will be the real vehicles that patients and providers alike will use to improve their health outcomes and lower their costs.

Many of the tools you will need to do this critical design work will come from the competitive and financial analyses previously outlined in Chapter 3, "Determining Your PSHP's Comprehensive Execution Strategy."

To get the greatest value out of your product planning efforts, we suggest always keeping three ideas in mind while designing your health plan's product offerings:

- Where your product fits in the current marketplace

- What specifications your ultimate payors require, e.g., commercial, Medicare and Medicaid

- The needs and preferences of your prospective consumers/members and the providers who will deliver your health plan's services

Failing to understand the needs of your prospective individual members and the providers who will deliver your health plan's services is a common pothole. While conducting a market demographic analysis, distributing surveys and holding focus groups can be a significant investment, this research ultimately will tell you what types of health plans will sell or are missing in your market — and that can help you determine the likely attractiveness of your products.

Analyzing your market demographics also can save you money. As discussed in Chapter 10, "Actuarial Considerations and Financial Management," actuaries use demographic, geographic, clinical and claims data — among other information — to make reasoned predictions that will help your plan prepare for the future. This includes calculating your members' collective risk score to identify the plan's insurance risk.

The reality is that no amount of fancy analytics will change the fact that your population's average risk score and its deviation from the norm is largely outside of your control. But there is good news. While you cannot directly control who enrolls in your plan, you can influence numerous factors that affect your population's health risk by how you design your plan's benefits (the features of your products). For example, you could lower monthly premiums for individuals who enroll and participate in smoking-cessation programs. You can also use targeted marketing techniques to try and get healthier members to enroll, such as sponsoring local 5K races.

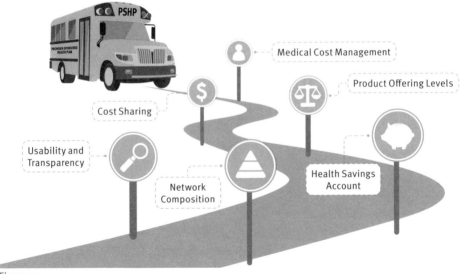

Key Factors of Plan Design
Source: Valence Health

Health plans construct their plan designs to satisfy their communities' unique needs and the organization's specialized mission. There are six key factors that will help determine the effectiveness of your plan design:

Figure 4.1

Medical Cost Management

Every individual consumer or member in your plan — young or old, man or woman, blue collar or white collar, chronically ill or healthy — has different medical needs and histories. Your PSHP can be more successful if it has product or plan features that address your specific population's medical needs and their care delivery preferences.

That said, your PSHP will first need to know what medical services (i.e., surgeries, prescriptions, physical therapy, etc.) are regularly being provided to your potential members. Your plan should also assess what recommended or preventative services seem to be missing from your population.

With this complete population-based healthcare utilization profile in hand, you can then begin to think about how your plan can help reduce the number of inappropriate or duplicative services and increase the amount of preventative or predictive services moving forward. By using a variety of medical management tools, your plan will aim to improve your members' health outcomes and reduce their medical costs (see Figure 4.2).

Common Medical Cost Management Tools
Source: Valence Health

- Clinical care guidelines or protocols for providers to use and follow when treating patients with certain conditions or risk factors
- Disease and condition management programs
- Patient engagement strategies such as support groups or the provision of personal medical devices for logging and reporting health information and/or vital signs

Figure 4.2

For example, maybe your local community has a large number of residents who have medical services associated with a lung cancer diagnosis or have a family history of lung cancer. The root cause for many of these patients may be smoking. So to counteract this population's health reality, your health plan can implement targeted smoking-cessation programs (or offer lower copays on smoking-cessation prescriptions and coupons for over-the-counter medications). Your PSHP's desire is to have these programs positively impact your members' health and reduce their need for costly healthcare services in the future.

One of the biggest struggles with improving population health is effectively engaging patients to follow recommended care guidelines. Now that you are fully at risk for the members in your plan, your PSHP is responsible for incentivizing them to use plan benefits in ways that will be the most beneficial for improving their collective health. Therefore, your medical cost management strategies become an extension and reinforcement of your PSHP's plan design. Involving your health plan's providers in planning any medical costs management efforts will also further ensure their success.

By creating the right clinical, support and condition management programs, as well as effective engagement strategies, you can help guide your patients toward a healthier way of life and better fulfill your mission as a healthcare organization.

Case Study:
Improving Population Health for Medicare Advantage Members with Medical Cost Management Strategies – *Kaiser Permanente*

Kaiser Permanente is the nation's largest and oldest provider-sponsored health plan, serving 10 million Americans in nine states. Kaiser Permanente of Colorado's (KPCO) 5-Star Medicare Advantage plan is on the leading edge of using patient-generated health data to drive innovative medical management programs for seniors and ultimately improve their care.

The PATHWAAY Program

In 2012, KPCO launched PATHWAAY – the Proactive Assessment of Total Health & Wellness to Aid Active Years – a primary care-based program to help seniors and physicians address tough topics during patient visits. Seniors are screened remotely prior to their wellness visits to unearth lifestyle risks that may keep them from being independent, e.g., risks for falls, urinary incontinence, malnutrition, pain, frailty and mood disorders.

Seniors first complete an online or telephonic total health assessment, describing symptoms, lifestyle choices and their health histories. Their answers flow into Kaiser's electronic health record, where the assessment is processed and scored for risk. Based on risk factors, some patients receive a follow-up call from a nurse, and all at-risk patients get a detailed, personalized prevention plan in their record. The plan is printed out during the member's annual wellness visit and used as a starting point for patient education.

Physicians say the program facilitates conversations about clinical issues that seniors hesitate to bring up. Patients say the prevention plans are easy to understand and follow. In a recent survey, more than 70 percent of participants said the program made them more confident in their ability to improve their health, and 57 percent reported taking action on their personal prevention plans.

The Health Bones Program

Nearly 15 years ago, Kaiser Permanente of Southern California (Kaiser SCAL) introduced its Healthy Bones program to proactively identify, screen and treat patients at risk for osteoporosis, falls and fractures.

With the help of information systems to identify at-risk patients and care gaps, case managers reach out to members to schedule bone density scans. Once complete, scan results are interpreted on the spot and given to patients. Some 40 percent of patients who get a scan qualify for treatment in the form of education (such as a fall prevention class); support (such as a home visit to assess fall risks); a prescription for exercise; and possibly medication. For every 100 patients enrolled in the program, Kaiser reports that one fewer hip fracture takes place.

In 2010 alone, the program's $5 million cost paid off ten-fold by preventing more than 1,000 hip fractures and saving roughly $40 million in surgery expenses. Because of Healthy Bones, Kaiser SCAL has been top-rated nationally among Medicare plans for osteoporosis management in women.

Sources: Kaiser presentations and publications from 2012–2015.

Additionally, your PSHP can design plans that encourage healthier individuals to enroll. For example, say your organization owns and operates a local health club. By creating plan incentives around buying and using a health club membership, you will attract members who either already use a health club or who are willing to begin using one. In general, this tends to be a healthier population group with a low actuarial risk that you can financially motivate to remain healthy with lower premiums.

Pricing: The Cost-Sharing Options You Use in Your PSHP's Plans

If your PSHP will be offering commercial products directly to employers or on an exchange, you also will have to compete on price. In fact, today, the price of available health plans is more critical than ever thanks to heightened transparency, increased consumerism and rising deductibles.

> **Expert Insight**
>
> *"Think about this: the first boxes you have to check off address your plan design and price points. If you are not competitive on price or design, you are not in the game. So those are your minimum requirements to compete."*
>
> **– Steve Cherok**
> Healthcare Vertical Practice Leader,
> Trion Group, A Marsh & McLennan Agency, LLC Company

When buying insurance products, both the ultimate payor and the individual member want to have the best pricing structure possible. For example, if the ultimate payor is an employer, then it wants to pay the most reasonable fees for each employee, including premium rates, administrative fees and stop-loss premiums. Individual members also want the best premium rates and least expensive cost-sharing options possible. Both health plan customers want to select the best plan available to them — both in terms of cost and quality.

If you have chosen to offer Medicare and/or Medicaid plans or products, the price the government will pay you for each enrolled member or service is set by a series of regulations. While there are definitely some factors that you can control, these factors will vary by state and service area. Therefore, you will need to specifically research what rules and regulations apply in your market. While all health plans have less flexibility in setting plan prices or reimbursement levels when the federal and/or state government are the ultimate payors, there are also countless PSHPs and other insurance companies that have financially successful Medicare and Medicaid plans.

All of these factors will help the executives in charge of pricing understand historic rates as well as future trends. Here is an important tip to keep in mind: do not underestimate the value of reading the newspaper or pulling your competitors' financial statements from last quarter. All of these are important elements to consider when setting your plan's prices (see Figure 4.3).

Primary Inputs for Setting Health Plan Prices

Source: Valence Health

- Your plan's past financial performance data
- Your competitors' past financial performance data
- Current events and general economic trends and conditions in your service area

Figure 4.3

The hardest part of this process will be pricing your products in the first year. Since you have likely never had health plans before, there is obviously no past performance data to analyze and learn from. Without this benchmark, the pricing process is definitely more challenging, but with thorough market research and the involvement of a good actuary, your PSHP can set competitive prices in year one. By the second year, this process will become easier as your organization will have experience to build on (for more information on plan pricing, refer to Chapter 10, "Actuarial Considerations and Financial Management").

A plan with both a sensible premium and financial incentives built into its benefit design will not only be appealing to the ultimate payor and the individual member, but also can enable you to better fulfill your mission as a healthcare provider. You can create health plan products that your members are not afraid to use because the out-of-pocket costs are too high or because certain services are severely limited. Your plan's members should feel comfortable going to the doctor because it can keep them healthier — and less expensive to insure — in the long run.

Plan Design Cost-Sharing Options: Deductibles, Copays and Coinsurance

Benefits design allows your PSHP to specify all the details of your plan's financial options. A key component of this is how medical expenses will be divided between the member and your PSHP. This plan component is called cost-sharing and is used in designing commercial, Medicare and Medicaid products.

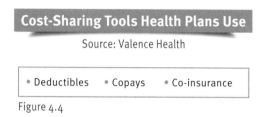

Figure 4.4

However, there are very specific rules around cost-sharing options for Medicare and Medicaid, so again you will have to study your owner's manual, i.e., federal and state regulations governing these programs. For example, with Medicaid, certain vulnerable groups, such as children and pregnant women, are exempt from most out-of-pocket costs and copayments. Keeping the ultimate payor in mind, you will have to define your plan's cost-sharing structure and establish the rules and dollar limits for all cost-sharing tools that you choose to use.

The deductible is a specified amount of money that the member must pay for healthcare services before the insurer, your organization, can begin paying any benefits. There are both individual deductibles, where the sole member pays the entire deductible, and family deductibles, in which the enrollee and their dependents count toward the total deductible amount. Regardless of the type of deductible, the fixed amount is set for a given benefit period — generally a year — and only applies to those services that your plan specifies.

As a PSHP, by strategically pricing and setting the rules around your plan's deductibles, you can effectively influence patient behavior. For example, many health plans are beginning to offer high-deductible health plans to promote more cost-conscious healthcare decision making and to make plans more affordable. The hope is that members will not misuse medical services, like going to the emergency department for something that might be best addressed in an outpatient office setting.

However, this becomes a delicate balancing act. Set the cost-sharing amounts associated with your plan correctly and with logical rules, and you can cut unnecessary healthcare spending. Set the cost-sharing amounts associated with your plan too high or have illogical rules, and members may be unable or unwilling to access necessary or preventative medical services, thereby increasing their future medical costs.

Health plans also use copay and coinsurance as cost-sharing mechanisms. Both of these are specific portions of the medical expenses that the members must pay themselves. However, one major difference is that copays are flat dollar amounts, while coinsurance is a percentage of the medical bill and will vary.

There are a number of different ways copays and coinsurance can be designed. Some Health Maintenance Organization (HMO) and Point of Service (POS) plans require copays without a deductible, while indemnity and Preferred Provider Organization (PPO) plans usually require coinsurance and a deductible. In fact, some plans do not even have copays. And while copays are typically collected at the time of service, some plans require copays for each inpatient admission, while others require one for every day of inpatient services.

The explanation of benefits (EOB), which your PSHP will have to create, is most often the rule book that has separate sections to address the copay and coinsurance amounts for all the plans you offer. Your EOB also must address copay amounts for outpatient versus inpatient services due to the cost differences associated with these service types.

Since PSHPs have more real-time access to their members' healthcare utilization trends, they are well-positioned to design plans that suit their various needs. If there is a large population that has high spending on prescription drugs, then a plan with low prescription copays will likely attract a higher number of enrollees. Likewise, maybe a plan with lots of elderly members will cover annual flu shots, even if the member has not reached his or her deductible.

Product Offerings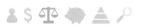

Now that you know the cost-sharing mechanisms for managing your organization's insurance risk, and the programs and engagement strategies for reducing medical costs, it is a matter of balancing these services and features with your plan's premium to create attractive products.

While consumers want the best insurance plan at the best price, they may forgo several optional services and features for those that are most important to them. Your plan needs to offer a fair price for the unique combination of plan services and features or otherwise consumers will look elsewhere.

To allow consumers to compare plans "apples to apples" or "bus to bus," many organizations categorize their insurance plans or products based upon their actuarial value, which is the average percentage of healthcare costs a health plan will cover. Plans with similar actuarial values are placed in the same plan level, or tiers, so consumers can more easily compare their options. While the terminology for these levels can vary for different organizations or marketplaces, the general concept remains the same.

The Affordable Care Act's "metallic tiers" model has become a popular example of this tiered structure. This model requires plans to be placed into one of four categories: platinum, gold, silver or bronze (see Figure 4.5). In the platinum or gold plans, the insurance company will cover more of the healthcare costs than in the silver and bronze plans. Therefore, the members' cost-sharing arrangements will be higher in the bronze and silver plans and lower in the gold and platinum plans, while members' premiums are the opposite. This tiered structure requires a plan's potential members to decide if it is more financially feasible for them to select inexpensive cost-sharing arrangements or lower premium rates.

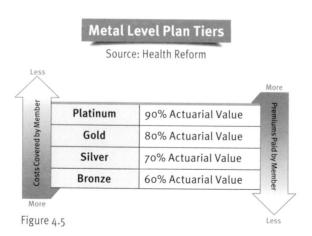

Figure 4.5

To provide enrollees with various options, your PSHP will need to go through an actuarial exercise that involves balancing the services and features of your plan's "bus." While you may want to offer Wi-Fi, roomy aisles and overhead reading lights, you may not need a TV, bathroom or full kitchenette.

If you add or remove any of these features, then you will need to balance it by making a comparable change, e.g., reducing or increasing the price of the bus pass. For example, if you increase the pharmacy benefit deductible, then you can add a complementary benefit where the first generic prescription is free. If you lower the number of services you cover by eliminating vision and dental coverage, then you can reduce the plan's premiums. In the end, your organization should tailor these combinations to the desires of your target market.

For example, maybe the young "invincible" population that rarely visits the doctor is searching for a bronze level plan with a low premium. Perhaps the working mother and father want a low family deductible with a wellness program, but do not need several services that generally are carved out or not included, like behavioral health. If you are offering a Medicare or Medicaid plan, you will have to follow a set of rules that dictate what services your plan must include and what you will have the freedom to adjust. In the end, your organization should tailor these combinations to the desired health outcomes and cost reductions you are hoping to achieve within your target market.

The key to designing a successful plan is to identify what your individual consumers both want and need, then deliver it in a way that encourages healthy behavior."

– Steve Tutewohl
Strategic Accounts Officer, Valence Health

Health Savings Accounts (HSAs)

One offering that some of your plan's individual members will want to ease their cost-sharing arrangements is a health savings account (HSA). An HSA is a tool that gives members more freedom and flexibility when deciding how to purchase and consume healthcare. If you offer an HSA benefit, they are typically selected by members at the time they enroll in your health plan. Individual members then have to select a total HSA dollar amount that will be deducted from the members' paychecks but are not taxed, so an HSA is considered tax-free benefit.

However, these tax-advantaged savings accounts are not for everyone. Typically associated with high-deductible plans, HSAs are designed to offset high out-of-pocket costs by allowing consumers to put aside or save pre-tax dollars to cover future medical costs. The intent of an HSA is to encourage smart healthcare choices and saving behaviors for those who generally have minimal healthcare expenses.

> ### Expert Insight
>
> *"Health savings accounts absolutely have a long-term place in the healthcare model of the future."*
>
> **– Jason Montrie**
> President, Land of Lincoln Health

Both the HSA's policyholder(s) and his or her employer can contribute money to the account, which accumulates over the years even if the individual switches employers. Individuals are generally encouraged to contribute regularly through payroll deductions or annual contributions. Although employers have no obligation to make contributions, many develop a contribution or matching component to facilitate the adoption of HSA plans or to encourage a healthier lifestyle. This can sometimes reduce the price of the overall health plans they select for their employees (see the case study, *Designing HSAs for Your Target Market* for an example).

Case Study:
Designing HSAs for Your Target Market – *MOBĒ, LLC*

"How you design your HSA makes a huge difference on which type of people will select your plan. For example, there is a plan that is designed to attract a healthier population in which we give the enrolled employees a pedometer. This device measures them on three different goals: how much they walk, how frequently they walk and whether they complete one long walk a day.

Then, the employer contributes to the employee's HSA $1 every day for each of the three predetermined goals they meet. So that is three goals a day, $3 a day, $90 a month and more than $1,000 a year that can potentially be contributed to the employee's HSA, depending on how much they walk! That is a very different health plan than one where the employer says, "If you select a high-deductible plan, I am going to give you $1,000."

Even though both of those HSAs are going to be targeted toward a younger and healthier population, adding a wellness program is a key design decision that can attract specific segments of the population."

– Gino Tenace
CEO, MOBĒ, LLC

Network Composition

Another way to influence member and provider behavior is by designing your plan's network to guide behavior. This involves contracting with medical professionals who offer services your PSHP will cover and then developing incentives that will motivate members to use certain physicians over others — namely, those who are in-network rather than out-of-network. To complement these patient incentives, many organizations also offer appropriate provider incentives for following clinical guidelines or care protocols and/or directing physicians' referral patterns toward in-network providers. As a result, your network is narrowed to better address members' health needs while managing costs.

To function properly, your plans must contract with a network of physicians and institutions that offer essential medical services and various specialties (see Figure 4.6). Through these contracts, your organization will establish a list of allowed charges, or discounted fees that reduce the cost of medical services. Those providers who are in-network agree through their contract to accept the allowed charges as full reimbursement. The range of value-based care incentives that your PSHP ultimately settles on will then be layered into your in-network reimbursement agreements (for more information on network development and contracts, refer to Chapter 6, "Network Development and Management").

The 10 Essential Health Benefits

Source: HealthCare.gov

When do you know if your provider network is complete? One good way to check is to look at the 10 essential health benefits. The Affordable Care Act developed these requirements as a way to ensure that plans sold on the state and federal exchanges provide all the core benefits that consumers should access to ensure better health outcomes. By critically evaluating your current network and assessing providers' ability to provide these benefits, your organization can ensure the plan's network is adequate.

If you choose to sell any of your PSHP's products or plans on the state and federal exchanges, you will have to offer these benefits in yours:

- Ambulatory patient services
- Emergency services
- Hospitalization
- Maternity and newborn care
- Mental health and substance use disorder services, including behavioral health treatment

- Prescription drugs
- Rehabilitative and habilitative services and devices
- Laboratory services
- Preventive and wellness services and chronic disease management
- Pediatric services, including oral and vision care

Figure 4.6

As your organization forms contracts with providers, hospitals and other healthcare providers, it can structure groups or tier providers (see Figure 4.7). These tiers are designed to guide members toward a group of narrower, in-network providers who have high-quality outcomes and who also have agreed to your plan's list of allowed charges and value-based care metrics. In effect, designing networks is another way your organization can influence where people receive their care.

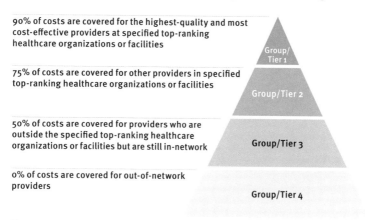

Sample Health Plan Group/Tier Structure

Source: Society for Human Resources Management and The Kroger Co.

90% of costs are covered for the highest-quality and most cost-effective providers at specified top-ranking healthcare organizations or facilities

Group/Tier 1

75% of costs are covered for other providers in specified top-ranking healthcare organizations or facilities

Group/Tier 2

50% of costs are covered for providers who are outside the specified top-ranking healthcare organizations or facilities but are still in-network

Group/Tier 3

0% of costs are covered for out-of-network providers

Group/Tier 4

Figure 4.7

To make narrow networks plans more impactful, your PSHP also can offer enhanced benefits. This means offering lower deductibles and copays, or maybe even extra incentives and clinical programs to offset the plan's more limited access to providers. With the addition of a coordinated patient care team, narrow networks plans can maintain quality, while minimizing costs.

If members would like to access a broader panel of providers, they can search within the plan's middle tiers of providers for a slightly higher cost. The lower tiers will cost more for members to access, but have little to no restrictions on providers that members can see (see the case study, *Tailoring Your Plan Design,* for an example). This tiered physician grouping or networking concept also encourages members to take more control of their well-being by selecting who they want to be able to access for their healthcare services before they purchase their health plan.

Case Study:

Tailoring Your Plan Design – *Land of Lincoln Health*

"In shaping our plans, Land of Lincoln Health created a unique plan design structure for network providers that we call three-tier plan designs. Tier one contains a group of preferred in-network physicians. Tier two has a broader network that contains our national representatives. And tier three contains providers who are out-of-network.

81

As you move up the tiers, the benefits continue to increase and the out-of-pocket costs are lower. If members do not go to your tier-one providers, you still have a good plan and they still have choice. We think that is a fundamental advantage for providers. In fact, that is how hospitals have been designing their own employees' benefits plans for years — placing themselves in tier one, a broader network in tier two and out-of-network in tier three.

Typically, hospitals that are large enough to contemplate this will have this type of plan design for their associates. We have found that most of those organizations see 80 percent to 85 percent of the care delivered to their own associates is funneled through their own system, since the plan design directs the members toward a specific set of providers. This means more benefits go to the sponsored organization and its affiliated physicians and specialists, making this plan design incredibly effective for the employees of these healthcare organizations."

– Jason Montrie
President, Land of Lincoln Health

Building Plan Design around Enhanced Usability and Transparency

Make your plan design intuitive.

Health insurance as a whole can be confusing, but when groups or individuals look at your products or plans, they need to understand what they are buying. In light of recent healthcare trends toward consumerism, your PSHP would be well-served by conducting some type of auditing process to ensure your plan's product offerings are easy to use and crystal clear to your average consumer. Remember, even though the ultimate payor and individual members tend to make their purchasing decisions based on price, they will not select a plan again if it was too difficult to understand or use. This means that all your communication vehicles — especially your EOB — should be something your target market can read, understand and easily navigate.

One way to do this is to simplify your plans. This is particularly important when looking at the different financial structures. Are your deductible, copay and coinsurance designs customer-friendly? For example, telling members they have a $20 copay for an MRI is much easier to understand than providing a coinsurance percentage for the same service.

Another way to do this is with transparency. Prospective members want to easily access and understand information about your plan's quality, cost and provider networks.

The National Committee for Quality Assurance (NCQA) has furthered the push for greater health plan transparency by introducing the Healthcare Effectiveness Data and Information Set (HEDIS) and the Consumer Assessment of Healthcare

Providers and Systems (CAHPS). These measures provide some objective means of evaluating health insurance organizations' clinical quality and patient satisfaction.

They, and similar metrics from other organizations, are designed to improve the value of healthcare by giving people the resources to critically compare their options. Consequently, these transparency measures also motivate healthcare professionals to improve their performance and demonstrate their commitment to quality to their patients.

By their very nature, PSHPs have an advantage in this area over more traditional health plans. Leadership throughout the PSHP and its affiliated providers can work together to improve physician quality, subsequently lowering medical costs and improving health outcomes. Likewise, it is relatively simple to determine which hospitals and physicians are affiliated with a PSHP as these organizations tend to be clearly linked to their parent company.

One obvious concern of prospective members is whether or not their current hospital and physicians are in-network. By addressing this concern upfront, individuals are more likely to select your potentially narrower local network over a broader, national network that is ambiguous about which local physicians are included. ⊘

Tracking Key Health Plan Design Metrics

Performing regular data analysis can help your PSHP maximize its return on investment and identify both early warning signs of trouble and indicators of success. By tracking key inputs and outputs, you can continually enhance your health plan so it retains members, remains financially stable and earns high patient satisfaction scores. Below are key plan design metrics that should be measured continuously:

- Plan's insurance risk, based upon your members' collective risk score
- Market studies, consumer surveys and focus groups to identify what sells or is missing in your marketplace
- Enrollee demographics (name, date of birth, gender, etc.)
- Enrollee medical conditions (diabetes, arthritis, high blood pressure, etc.)
- Enrollee treatment information (medications, surgeries, physical therapy, etc.)
- Public health data for your service area

- Risk management strategies
- Cost-sharing arrangements
- Medical cost management strategies
- Plan pricing and offerings
- Network size, providers and contracts
- Your plan's past financial and operational performance
- Competitors' past financial and operational performance data
- HSA enrollment
- Plan usability and transparency metrics
- HEDIS and CAHPS score

Industry Terminology Related to Plan Design

Actuarial Risk   A statistical method of estimating the risk of a particular event's occurrence (e.g., the risk of inpatient hospital admission). Actuarial methods are touted as more accurate than clinical judgment alone.

Source: Valence Health

Actuarial Value   The percentage of total average costs for covered benefits that a plan will cover. For example, if a plan has an actuarial value of 70%, on average, you would be responsible for 30% of the costs of all covered benefits. However, you could be responsible for a higher or lower percentage of the total costs of covered services for the year, depending on your actual healthcare needs and the terms of your insurance policy.

Source: HealthCare.gov

Administrative Fees   Payment for those business expenses that health plans incur when managing the non-clinical aspects of your health plan, e.g., printing membership cards, personnel and systems related to provider and member customer service portals, or overhead expenses.

Source: Valence Health

Coinsurance   The patient's share of the costs for a covered healthcare service, calculated as a percent (for example, 20%) of the allowed amount for the service. The member pays coinsurance plus any deductibles they may owe. For example, if the health insurance or plan's allowed amount for an office visit is $100 and the patient met the deductible, his coinsurance payment of 20% would be $20. Your health insurance plan pays the rest of the allowed amount.

Source: HealthCare.gov

Consumer Assessment of Healthcare Providers and Systems (CAHPS)   Surveys that ask consumers and patients to report on and evaluate their experiences with healthcare. These surveys focus on aspects of quality that consumers are best qualified to assess, such as the communication skills of providers and ease of access to healthcare services.

Source: Agency for Healthcare Research and Quality

Copay   A fixed amount (for example, $15) the member pays for a covered healthcare service, usually when the service is delivered. The amount also can vary by the type of covered healthcare service. Outpatient office visits may have a $25 copay, while emergency room visits could have a $150 copay.

Source: HealthCare.gov

Deductible   The amount patients owe for healthcare services before their health insurance or plan begins to pay. For example, if your deductible is $1,000, your plan will not cover anything until you have paid that full amount. The deductible, however, may not apply to all services. For example, an annual physical will be paid for regardless if you have spent $1,000 on other covered services.

Source: HealthCare.gov

Explanation of Benefits (EOB)   A statement sent by a health insurance company to covered individuals explaining what medical treatments and/or services were paid for on their behalf.

Source: Valence Health

Health Maintenance Organization (HMO)   A type of health insurance plan that usually limits coverage to care from doctors who work for or contract with the HMO. It generally will not cover out-of-network care except in an emergency. An HMO may require you to live or work in its service area to be eligible for coverage. HMOs often provide integrated care and focus on prevention and wellness.

Source: HealthCare.gov

Health Savings Account (HSA)   A medical savings account available to taxpayers who are typically enrolled in a high-deductible health plan. The funds contributed to the account are not subject to federal income tax at the time of deposit. Funds must be used to pay for qualified medical expenses. Funds roll over year to year if they are not spent.

Source: HealthCare.gov

Healthcare Effectiveness Data and Information Set (HEDIS)   A tool used by more than 90% of America's health plans to measure performance on important dimensions of care and service. Altogether, HEDIS consists of 81 measures across five domains of care. Because so many plans collect HEDIS data, and because the measures are so specifically defined, HEDIS makes it possible to compare the performance of health plans on an "apples-to-apples" basis.

Source: National Committee for Quality Assurance

Indemnity Plan   A type of health plan under which a covered person must pay 100% of all covered charges up to the plan's annual deductible. Once the deductible is met, a percentage of the covered charges must be paid by the covered person, up to the plan's out-of-pocket maximum. Indemnity plans do not usually offer in- or out-of-network benefit restrictions, but out-of-pocket costs are usually less when services are received by in-network healthcare professionals.

Source: Cigna.com/glossary

Medical Management An umbrella term that includes utilization management, case management and disease management functions. Medical management strategies and programs are designed to improve population health by guiding consumer and/or provider behavior toward the healthiest options. Also synonymous with Medical Cost Management.

Source: Valence Health

Point of Service (POS) A type of plan in which you pay less if you use doctors, hospitals and other healthcare providers that belong to the plan's network. POS plans also require you to get a referral from your primary care doctor in order to see a specialist.

Source: HealthCare.gov

Preferred Provider Organization (PPO) A type of health plan that contracts with medical providers, such as hospitals and doctors, to create a network of participating providers. You pay less if you use providers that belong to the plan's network. You can use doctors, hospitals and providers outside of the network for an additional cost.

Source: HealthCare.gov

Premium The amount that must be paid by the insured for his/her health insurance or plan. The member or his/her employers usually pay the premium monthly, quarterly or yearly.

Source: HealthCare.gov

Risk Score In a typical health risk assessment, each individual is scored based on an algorithm that incorporates information on the individual's age, any illnesses during the previous year and other factors. Patients' responses to health questions generate a numerical value, which is combined to produce a risk score so that a weighted average value can be determined and used to compare the relative risk of one population to another.

Source: Actuary.com

Stop-Loss Premium The dollar amount of claims filed for eligible expenses at which point you have paid 100% of your out-of-pocket and the insurance begins to pay at 100%. Stop-loss is reached when an insured individual has paid the deductible and reached the out-of-pocket maximum amount of coinsurance.

Source: Healthinsurance.org

Chapter Five

Sales and Marketing

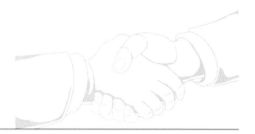

Now that your provider-sponsored health plan (PSHP) has products that are potentially better than any other plans in your market, your next big step is to make sure the predominant payors agree with you. If no one buys your plans or realizes their value, your PSHP will not be serving its purpose, meeting its objectives or fulfilling its mission. That is why sales and marketing is an essential function for your new PSHP. Ultimately, well-thought-out and executed sales and marketing capabilities will help attract target members.

Sales and Marketing Considerations by Payor/Line of Business

Source: Valence Health

Payor	Sales and Distribution Channels	Marketing Considerations*
Commercial	• Via brokers, for employer-sponsored health insurance • Direct to employers • Direct to members for public and private exchanges • Direct to individuals who are not on an exchange	• Involves business-to-business (B2B) and business-to-consumer (B2C) marketing strategies and tactics
Medicare	• Direct to members for Medicare Advantage	• Involves B2C marketing strategies and tactics • Must comply with all relevant Centers for Medicare & Medicaid Services (CMS) guidelines

Medicaid	• Differs state by state, but can include:
	  – Responding to and winning requests for proposals
	  – Receiving members via auto-enrollment by the state Medicaid agency
	  – Direct to members
	  – Via brokers who act on behalf of the state Medicaid agency
		• Involves B2B and B2C marketing strategies and tactics
		• Must comply with all relevant CMS and state Medicaid agency guidelines

*Governed by all relevant Health Insurance Portability and Accountability Act (HIPPA) and other healthcare privacy rules and regulations		

Figure 5.1

While sales and marketing might seem intuitive, there also are nuances in the health insurance business that deserve further explanation and consideration. Most notably, there will be a number of different health insurance regulations about marketing that you will have to follow. These rules will vary by state, and depending on the types of products you are selling will impact how you can market your plans to providers and/or members. To use our bus analogy, if you start driving at night without your lights on, your PSHP will be much more likely to hit a few bumps in the road.

Selling Your Plan: Knowing What Distribution Channel You Need to Master

As Figure 5.1 illustrates, how you deliver your health plan to your prospective members depends on the payors you are targeting. With this line-of-business lens in mind, your PSHP can sell specifically to:

- Employers via brokers or directly via their executive teams

- Individuals, both on and off public and private exchanges

- Government agencies, e.g., Medicare and Medicaid

Common Sales Tactics Used to Build Broker Relationships

Source: Valence Health

- Hold education meetings with members of your local broker community
- Prepare employer-centric customized materials and data that address your unique:
  - Healthcare services
  - Medical cost management strategies
  - Health outcomes for similar populations of employees
- Analyze your plan's pricing options* in advance of any initial discussion or negotiation

*For more information on pricing see Chapter 4, "Plan Design"

Figure 5.2

Employer Sales

If your health plan offers a commercial product, employers that directly offer health insurance to their employees are your key sales prospects. In many cases, reaching employers requires your plan's sales team to work with and convince independent brokers about the value of your plan(s). In other instances, you may want to work directly with an employer's executive team.

Like in other types of insurance, healthcare brokers represent their clients' best interests. Their job is to work with plans like yours to find the best option that will deliver the best return on investment (ROI) for the employers they serve. Brokers can also be an added channel for marketing your PSHP and increasing awareness of your products. As you can probably tell, building a good relationship with these brokers is critical to your health plan's success. So how can you use brokers effectively?

Brokers and the companies they represent want to find the best products available, so it is your PSHP's responsibility to convince them you have the better bus (see Figure 5.2). Whether you are dealing with a broker or the employer directly, you will want to leverage your value proposition and any supporting data you gathered when conducting your market analysis as part of your sales pitch (refer to the Understanding Payor Competition and Concentration section in Chapter 3, "Determining Your PSHP's Comprehensive Execution Strategy").

You also will want to highlight any services and features that could be attractive to the employees who ultimately will be covered by your PSHP. For example, does your plan allow online bill payment for tech-savvy members? Is your customer service center open at times that would be convenient for employees who work shifts?

If you create meaningful alignment between your PSHP's offering and the employer's workforce — and can communicate that value — you will have a much more meaningful sales conversation. For more information about working with brokers, see the case study, *Using Brokers to Help Sell Your PSHP's Value Proposition*.

A number of our clients are taking greater control of their commercial full-risk arrangements by working directly with employer executives from the very start. They are:

- Designing and simultaneously selling health plans specifically for that employer's workforce and their beneficiaries

- Forming networks of providers and health plan features by appropriately leveraging the employer's historical employee healthcare data and information

- Bringing services directly into the workplace with things like work-site urgent care facilities

As your PSHP thinks about working with employers, know that their interest in your health plan may vary depending on the size of their employee population and their method of structuring health insurance plans. From the employer's vantage point, there are two common forms of insurance products: fully insured or self-insured health plans.

Case Study:
Using Brokers to Help Sell Your PSHP's Value Proposition — *Aon*

"Brokers' interactions have traditionally taken the form of broker-to-payor, as they represent their clients. However, brokers are increasingly looking at direct contracting vehicles with providers.

As an example, it would be compelling for brokers to tell their client they have a plan option available with a vetted health system that performs a high volume of musculoskeletal procedures (e.g. things like total and partial hip and knee replacements) with a low readmission rate. A corporation with a high density of musculoskeletal issues for their employees in that same geographic area might consider directing flow to a healthcare organization like this.

Brokers also need to convey the providers' ease of access and ease of use. Once you have proven to the client that the proposed healthcare system drives consistently good clinical results, you will also need to know if employees can quickly access the system and see the types of physicians they need.

With these two pieces of information in hand, the healthcare provider can approach the employer and say, 'We want to provide care for your patients. Let's work out a center of excellence around musculoskeletal issues at a referenced-based price and get more of your employees to think about going there.'

Effectively selling your health plan requires learning about the segments of your target populations and figuring out if you have a good value proposition for them."

– Matthew Levin
Executive Vice President and Head of Global Strategy, Aon

Fully insured health plans are the more traditional method of health plan structuring. These health plans bear the risk associated with offering health insurance and collect monthly premiums from the employer to pay healthcare claims. This method is usually more attractive to small employers because it evens out the dollars associated with unknown claims. Regardless of the employees' fluctuating medical bills, the employer will have predictable costs related to paying for health insurance on a monthly basis.

Understanding Why Employers Also Use Stop-Loss Insurance

Source: Valence Health

While your PSHP will have its stop-loss insurance, the employers that contract with your plan will likely carry their own polices. Why?

If an employer's healthcare claims are more expensive than anticipated, this can place the company in a financially challenging position. For this reason, employers also use stop-loss insurance to cover healthcare expenses that exceed expected levels.

Figure 5.3

In contrast, large employers often use a self-insured health plan in which they assume the risk of providing healthcare coverage. The chief financial officers (CFOs) or other executives in these companies are frequently interested in pursuing creative or new options for controlling healthcare costs. By acting as their own insurer, these companies take the premium dollars that would have been paid to an external health plan and use those funds to pay claims instead.

Selecting the Sales Pitch for Employer Health Plans

When selling your commercial plan to employers, you have three main parties to please: human resources (HR), consultants and the CFO. While HR executives often function as the buyer and face of the corporation when you are trying to sell your PSHP, simply know that they are not always the decision makers. As with any good sales plan, make sure your PSHP's sales team has drawn out some sort of a unique decision matrix for each party it deals with.

To win over HR (and any consultants that are influencing its decision), there are two important points to keep in mind. First, HR's baseline concern is that your plan satisfies its minimum benefit requirements. Second, it is critical to keep in mind that one of HR's key functions is to help resolve employees' complaints about their healthcare. Therefore, your sales pitch for employee-focused products should include proof points that show how your plan reduces insurance-related complaints and makes HR executives' lives easier.

When dealing with the CFO, your sales messages should center on your plan's fiscal responsibility and proven ability to lower healthcare costs. Be warned that the primary challenge will be reaching the CFO to get a meeting at all. While CFOs are more involved in selecting their employees' health insurance than ever before — especially those who are interested in self-insured plans — they still are in many cases less involved than they should be.

As your plan competes for the attention and approval of HR and the CFO, you can expect the employer's incumbent health insurance company to join the discussion. If your plan beats the incumbent's price, it is common for HR to ask the incumbent to lower its prices. Of course, the incumbent will not want to lose business, so it will generally offer premium relief to keep itself in business. Knowing that this pricing dance might happen and being prepared to offer alternatives is something successful PSHPs are well prepared for.

Have you ever paid cash when you rode the bus and told the driver to keep the change? Even though you are taking a hit financially, you realize waiting for change simply is not worth the hassle. The same principle holds true during health insurance contract negotiations when employers seek to switch carriers. While incumbents might not lower their price to match yours exactly, they may get within 2, 3 or 4 percent of it. At that point, the aggravation cost to the corporation, or the hassle of switching carriers, overrides any financial savings.

Remember, although larger employers historically have tended to contract with national health plans, your PSHP's unique value proposition and medical management initiatives may motivate them to work with you, especially if they have an employee base that is largely located in your service area.

Individual Consumer Sales – On and Off Exchanges

When consumers shop for health plans on state and federal exchanges, they can only see the bare bones of each plan. As with any industry, the individual consumer's decision to buy your PSHP often boils down to price. And who could blame them? For this reason, it is critical that you promote your plan as affordable on exchanges — at least in the immediate future. You can certainly bolster your exchange presence via targeted marking, and we will address those tactics in the "Marketing Your PSHP" section later in this chapter.

In addition to the public exchanges, major consulting firms and other market surveys predict that 20 percent to 33 percent of employers will adopt private exchanges by 2017[1]. Therefore, if employers in your PSHP's market have already made this move, your PSHP will be in a dual-sales situation. First, your plan will have to make sure it is listed on any private exchange and second, your commercial products will have to appeal directly to the healthcare needs and preferences of the employees who are purchasing their healthcare in this similar marketplace.

For individuals who do not meet public exchange eligibility requirements and do not have employer health insurance, there is an individual purchasing market (see Figure 5.4). This same pricing approach needs to be taken with any direct individual sales efforts your plan pursues. Ensuring that all individual plans are in sync with one another is a hallmark of successful healthcare insurance companies. If these consumers already know your brand or have seen your marketing campaigns, they may want to work with your health plan directly to enroll in one of its products. Under these circumstances, your best sales strategy may be to prominently display the plan on your PSHP's website to route prospective members to plan options, applications and enrollment instructions.

---

1 Resilience.willis.com/articles/2014/04/25/how-private-exchanges-are-reshaping-us-healthcare/

Factors Impacting Individual Health Plan Purchasing

Source: Valence Health

Select Affordable Care Act (ACA) Exchange Exclusion Criteria	Examples of Individual Health Plan Purchasers
• Individuals earning more than $46,680 annually • Consumers living in states that do not have public exchanges	• Full-time freelancers • Senior executives in limited liability corporations who are not covered by the company's health insurance, e.g., partners in some law and consulting firms

Figure 5.4

Some of Valence Health's PSHP clients also use partners to help them manage their individual on and off-exchange sales. Typically, this means your PSHP's prospective members will be directed to the vendor's website storefront or to the exchanges if they are eligible and are searching for health insurance.

Government Sales

While it sounds somewhat backward to say your health plan may have to sell its products to Medicare and Medicaid, there are things you have to do to be deemed eligible to sell your plans to individuals who are covered by these payors. There are various applications, requests for proposals and other requirements you will have to complete and be approved for before you can even begin.

If approved, your sales tactics will be heavily regulated by CMS and/or a state's Medicaid agency. However, once that approval is in place, your sales tactics may mimic what you are doing for other payors. For example, Medicare Advantage (MA) plans are sold directly to individual MA-eligible members in defined geographic areas. Therefore, if your PSHP offers an MA product, this sales process will largely replicate what you do for individual consumer sales.

As Figure 5.1 illustrates, a PSHP's options for Medicaid sales differ greatly from state to state. Depending on what your local rules and regulations are (like in those states where the state Medicaid agency automatically enrolls Medicaid-eligible members in certain approved health plans), you may not need any Medicaid sales capabilities or tactics.

No matter whom you sell your PSHP's products to, there are instances when each and every major payor group issues a request for proposal (RFP). If you are interested in winning that business, know that some of your sales capabilities will need to be focused on being able to collect and present complex data and information.

In short, you will need great researchers and writers who understand the wants and needs of the payors who issue the RFPs. How you choose to handle your RFP sourcing and completion needs will be another build, buy and partner/outsource decision, which we address at length in Chapter 3, "Determining Your PSHP's Comprehensive Execution Strategy."

Benchmarking and Considerations for a PSHP's Sales and Marketing Function

Sources: 2013 Sherlock Company Baseline Review, 2013 Health Insurance Industry Sales Force Compensation Survey, HR+Survey Solutions, Valence Health

	Health Insurance Sales	Health Insurance Marketing
Critical Executive Skill Sets	• Broker experience • Government agency experience	• Combined B2B and B2C experience • Knowledge of CMS Marketing Guidelines, if applicable
	• Combined healthcare and insurance industry knowledge and experience • Network management and/or managed care contracting knowledge and experience	
Departmental Budget Considerations	• 12,000 members per sales employee	• The ACA created the 80/20 Medical Loss Ratio rule, with 20% of premiums being allowed for administrative costs
Execution Considerations	• 70% of companies use sales bonuses and more than 50% use commissions to motivate their sales teams	• A 2013 spending analysis of 16 PSHPs indicated that sales and marketing PMPM expenses were 4.4% of total administrative costs
	• Build, buy or partner/outsource consideration as outlined in Chapter 3, "Determining Your PSHP's Comprehensive Execution Strategy."	

Figure 5.5

Marketing Your PSHP

From a marketing standpoint, successful PSHPs position their organizations as an extension of their provider network. In learning from their efforts, your PSHP should aim to have all of its marketing programs reinforce the key points of differentiation that your plan has created and believes it can build its future reputation on. Your PSHP also requires solid marketing ideas and great execution that distinguishes your product from the competition. You need to insert your name and value proposition into this already crowded space using creative marketing campaigns.

Expert Insight

"When you study the provider-sponsored health plans that have successfully transitioned into becoming both a provider and a health plan, it starts very local. I think brand is important because that local member base is already full of customers. It's key that my patients can become my future members, and hopefully my brand as a health system and health plan matters in that decision."

– Steve Cherok
Healthcare Vertical Practice Leader,
Trion Group, A Marsh & McLennan Agency, LLC Company

As a brand new PSHP, you will likely need to leverage the brand awareness and perceived quality of the affiliated healthcare organizations that are part of your plan before you introduce an insurance product in your community. Your marketing team's task is to determine how you can reinforce the public's perception of your affiliated provider organization and transfer that sentiment to your new health plan (see Figure 5.5).

Part of the marketing team's job in any health plan is to communicate the plan's clinical, community and cost-reduction improvements. Seeing that the providers who formed and joined your plan's network are also deeply invested in local population health activities, your plan will have an endless source of marketing content.

Case Study:
Medical Management is Also Marketing

As a PSHP, your ability to deliver superior clinical outcomes at lower costs will be the theme in all of your marketing messages. Therefore, anything your plan does to engage the community and creatively encourage health behavior is like riding a triple decker bus. It is a great ride for patients, for providers and for marketers.

Scott & White Health Plan serves more than 200,000 members across 50 counties in central Texas. The plan's RightCare program for Medicaid patients is taking patient engagement to a new level by holding frequent focus groups with both members and care managers. This direct feedback then gets turned into innovative programs, including:

- **Smoking-cessation:** The plan's "Clearing the Air" program starts with care managers asking members if they want help quitting tobacco products. If members agree to be under physician care for smoking-cessation, they can choose from an expanded list of medications and products not on the Medicaid formulary to help them quit at no cost.

- **Free car seat installation:** Members who have had at least four prenatal visits are eligible for a free infant car seat and installation by certified technicians, along with instruction on car seat safety. With enough well-child visits, the member can later receive a free toddler car seat. By staying current with early childhood visits and immunizations, members can receive a free child booster seat.

- **Unlimited health-related calls and texting:** RightCare members ages 18 or older can receive cell phones where all health-related calls and texts are free. It is a great way to reach members without computers to share appointment reminders and healthcare guidance.

Source: Lynn, George. "Empowering Board Members to Improve Population Health through Value-Based Care." American Hospital Associations' Center for Healthcare Governance. 2014.

Like every other functional area in your PSHP, the marketing department will have to live with a budget and set up metrics that will help everyone on your PSHP's leadership team understand what resulted from your various marketing efforts. Therefore, as you make your plan's marketing content and channel decisions, you will have to make a series of trade-off decisions that are aligned with the products, payors and customers you have targeted.

For example, if your PSHP is going to offer commercial products on a public exchange, you will want to make marketing choices that reinforce how your plan's prospective members:

- Research and choose their health plans

- Perceive your plan's brand

- Value specific incentives

- Are willing to spend on their healthcare (given certain services)

- Are loyal to their current physicians

- Care about health plan transparency and usability

Since you will not be able to fund all of your potential marketing activities, be sure to think about how you can appropriately tap into your plan's provider network to become an extension of your marketing team. For example, doctors and hospitals in your plan can help you increase awareness by using their existing forums to market your plan through lunch-and-learns, educational webinars or other community-based activities. These marketing strategies can go a long way in helping to establish your health plan as an option your local target market will trust over a national insurance company.

Health plan marketing sits at a very unique intersection as it can be deeply personal and complicated (see Figure 5.6). Your PSHP will have all the same communication vehicles and tactical marketing options available to them as any other industry. Your plan can have a Facebook page, sponsor a softball team and write press releases (see Figure 5.6). On any given day, your target market could be the CEO of your area's largest employer, the nurses in a doctor's office, and the teachers at your local elementary school and their families (for examples of health plan marketing initiatives, see the case study, *Innovative Marketing Practices for PSHPs*).

What's Not Different About PSHP Marketing	What Is Different About PSHP Marketing
Just like a local car dealership or restaurant, your PSHP can access any marketing channel available in the broader community: • Paid advertising • Social media • Websites • Electronic and printed collateral • Direct mail campaigns to target members • Hosting events – like health fairs	Because you are a healthcare provider, an insurance company and have access to personal health information, portions of your PSHP's marketing will be regulated; e.g.: • Not disclosing patients' names when relating health outcomes and success stories • Submitting enrollment marketing materials to CMS or the state Medicaid agency for approval before using

Source: Valence Health
Figure 5.6

Case Study:
Innovative Marketing Practices for PSHPs

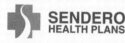 "Texas-based Sendero Health Plans recently introduced two mascots, Chips and Star, to promote STAR, Texas' Medicaid-managed care plan, and the Children's Health Insurance Program (CHIP) to entice Medicaid enrollees to enroll in these health plans. This initiative incorporates videos and other content directed at educating children and families on key health issues, ultimately with the aim of establishing brand affinity and loyalty."

 "AmeriHealth Caritas, a national PSHP, is committed to working with providers and community organizations to tackle important children's health issues, such as asthma and obesity. Its Healthy Hoops program involves more than 8,000 children and families. It features basketball clinics for children to learn hands-on asthma and obesity management skills that are taught by local and regional basketball legends. Healthy Hoops is one of the most comprehensive intervention programs available, recognized by the National Committee for Quality Assurance (NCQA) and America's Health Insurance Plans (AHIP) for innovation and leadership."

UPMC HEALTH PLAN "The UPMC Health Plan utilizes the latest approaches in social media – from its dedicated YouTube channel to a rich content resource in its UPMC MyHealthMatters blog – to reach potential members with educational information and insights. These approaches position UPMC as more than just a provider or a health plan, but as a valued partner in healthy living."

As a combined marketing and sales team, you will be accountable for communicating your PSHP's value proposition and brand value to the right individuals. Together, you will have to generate new business and watch what your competitors are doing. You often will be asked to reflect your customers' wants and needs so that your PSHP can innovate and evolve — explore new bus routes — while keeping your members and providers highly satisfied. ⊘

Tracking Key Health Plan Sales and Marketing Metrics

Performing regular data analysis can help your PSHP maximize its return on investment and identify both early warning signs of trouble and indicators of success. By tracking key inputs and outputs, you can continually enhance your health plan so it retains members, remains financially stable and earns high patient satisfaction scores. Below are key sales and marketing metrics that should be measured continuously:

- Number of new business leads
- Size of local employers' employee population
- Number of targeted employers with fully insured or self-insured health plans
- Medicare and Medicaid regulation changes
- Health insurance exchange regulation changes
- Enrollee demographics (name, date of birth, gender, etc.)
- Healthcare organization's patient satisfaction and Hospital Consumer Assessment of Healthcare Providers and Systems scores
- Potential member population size
- Actual member enrollment
- Plan rates
- Member satisfaction information
- Provider satisfaction information
- Marketing effectiveness metrics, e.g., website visitors, media coverage
- Brand awareness over time

Industry Terminology Related to Sales and Marketing

Brokers   An insurance broker sells, solicits or negotiates insurance for compensation.

Source: Valence Health

Carriers   A commercial enterprise licensed in a state to sell insurance.

Source: Valence Health

Medical Management   An umbrella term that includes utilization management, case management and disease management functions. Medical management strategies and programs are designed to improve population health by guiding consumer and/or provider behavior toward the healthiest options. Also synonymous with Medical Cost Management.

Source: Valence Health

Premium   The amount that must be paid by the insured for his/her health insurance or plan. The member or his/her employers usually pay the premium monthly, quarterly or yearly.

Source: HealthCare.gov

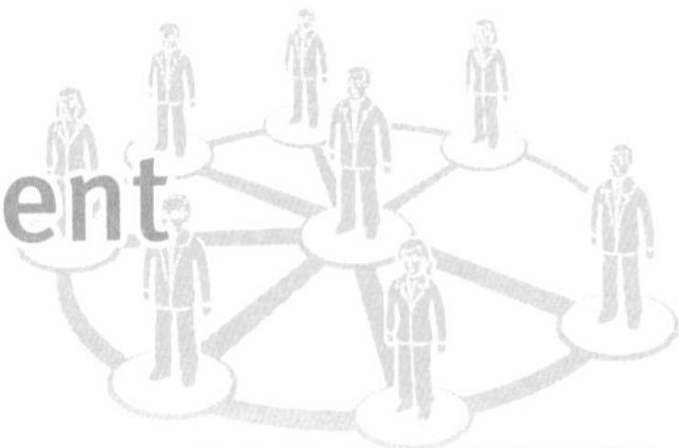

Chapter Six

Network Development and Management

When health plans refer to "network development" and "network management," they are specifically talking about aligning a group of healthcare practitioners and institutions that will provide healthcare services to the plan's members. Traditionally, people think of networks as providers and the hospitals in which they work, but they also include healthcare services like physical therapy and other ancillary functions offered by skilled nursing facilities, chiropractic clinics, etc. For a provider-sponsored health plan (PSHP), this includes all the providers under contract who offer care to your plan's populations.

Another Value-Based Care Model: The Clinically Integrated Network (CIN)

Source: Valence Health

While you have chosen to become a PSHP, other organizations you may choose to contract with may be part of a CIN already. Unlike the hospital networks of old that interacted with doctors to drive referrals back to the hospital and fill beds, today's CINs are very different.

CINs bring together numerous institutions, employed and independent doctors to really manage healthcare costs and quality. To be recognized as a CIN by the Federal Trade Commission, the network must establish and follow quality guidelines and monitor providers' performance — including eliminating those who are unable to meet agreed-upon standards. In return for doing this, CINs can contract directly with payors or health insurance organizations like your PSHP.

Figure 6.1

Defining Your Network's Needs

A key part of developing and managing a provider network lies in figuring out what medical services your plan's owners want to offer members. However, while you would never allow just any mechanic to work on your bus, you similarly do not want just any provider in your network — you want the best ones available that make sense for your plan. That said, as a PSHP, you will begin by assessing your affiliated healthcare providers as you develop your network (see Figures 6.1 and 6.2). Then you will want to recruit the top-performing providers you most want and need.

 For more information on blue highlighted text, refer to industry terminology at the end of the chapter.

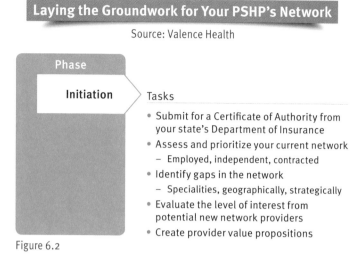

Figure 6.2

No matter what organizations come together to form your PSHP — a hospital and a large independent physician group, six independent physician groups or one integrated network — you will need to take a hard look at the network created by your plan's ownership structure. As a collection of healthcare practitioners, what are the group's strengths and weaknesses in terms of providers, services, quality and costs?

You need to be brutally honest with yourself at this point: does the network have all that is required to successfully operate the PSHP "bus"? In all likelihood, this will not be the case, so at the very least, you will need to contract with other providers who do not work for your affiliated hospitals or employed physician groups to close some network gaps.

Convincing providers to join and remain in your network is something that PSHPs and insurers nationwide deal with on a daily basis. Your PSHP will need to make strong efforts to entice providers by offering an appealing combination of patient volume and incentives for the least amount of hassle.

It also is very important to understand providers' unique points of view toward a provider network. Hospitals, physicians and ancillary service providers all will have their own opinions and concerns. Taking this feedback into consideration will be critical to your success; everyone involved needs to feel like they have a real stake in the game. But as long as they find value for their patients and themselves in what your PSHP offers, most providers should be willing to discuss the possibility of joining your network and forging a mutually beneficial relationship.

Expert Insight

"When forming contracts with prospective providers or facilities, you need to intentionally forge mutually beneficial relationships. These partnerships are a practical way to ensure network stability, but they do not occur by chance. Your PSHP needs to actively reach out to prospective providers and facility leadership to foster those relationships.

By developing contractual agreements with meaningful incentive programs, your PSHP can effectively encourage and reward providers who achieve specific levels of quality care, service and efficiency that benefit all stakeholders."

– J.C. McWilliams
System Vice President of Managed Care and Network Management,
Dean Health Plan

As with most things, you will probably want to have some options to choose from. It is likely that you will not want to include every provider in your PSHP's network and that you will want to partner with some external providers. When screening prospective providers, you will want to base some of your choices on the providers' geographic coverage (see Figure 6.3), subjective reputation and quantitative quality data.

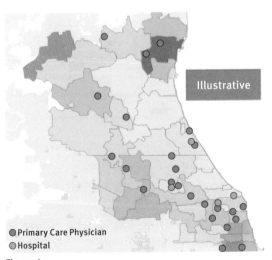

Figure 6.3

The primary concern with identifying prospective providers for your network should be access and quality. Your members need to be able to easily access all of your services without having to travel too far.

Typically, this is not an issue for most of the services your members will want to access because most of your network providers will be familiar, trusted members of the local community. Likewise, to form a well-rounded network, you have to contract with a diverse group of providers who have availability to take on new patients and offer non-traditional hours. The lack thereof may be a red flag.

This is where network development plays a huge role. When working to include some of the services you lack, but that your members will likely need and want, you have to determine the location and hours of these providers. Having a great radiology function will not mean much to your members if they have to drive an hour each way to get a CT scan during work hours.

Equally important is a prospective provider's reputation for quality care, given both subjective and objective data. This valuable information can be gathered by simply asking your prospective members or your affiliated health plan's physicians and leadership about whom they would and would not like to have in-network. This feedback can complement more objective sources of quality data. The Centers for Medicare and Medicaid Services (CMS) and the Agency for Healthcare Research and Quality (AHRQ) are just two publicly available sources that provide quantitative measures around providers' clinical quality, efficiency and service (see Figure 6.4). Once your PSHP contracts with providers, it will collect and analyze its own quantitative and qualitative data to assure the plan has the right providers in its network.

Although it may cost more initially to have exceptional providers join your network, the potential ability to then publicize the reputation of your PSHP may be worth the extra costs. You may also need to include a larger number of these "premium" providers in order to woo commercial employers that want to tout the quality of care they are offering their employees by working with your PSHP.

The prospective providers and facilities also must be filtered through your health plan's credentialing process. This thorough screening has rules and standards that are designed to separate quality providers who satisfy the plan's requirements from lower-quality providers, especially those with grievous sanctions, suspensions, or pending and completed malpractice suits. Therefore, it is critical that your credentialing standards are well-vetted and meet state and federal requirements — along with those of any local applicable accrediting bodies.

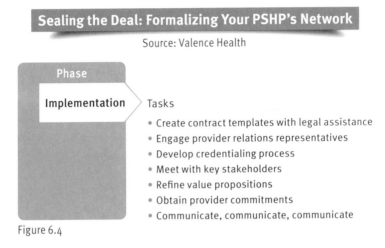

Sealing the Deal: Formalizing Your PSHP's Network

Source: Valence Health

Phase

Implementation

Tasks

- Create contract templates with legal assistance
- Engage provider relations representatives
- Develop credentialing process
- Meet with key stakeholders
- Refine value propositions
- Obtain provider commitments
- Communicate, communicate, communicate

Figure 6.4

Network adequacy is another regulatory requirement that your health plan must address through network development. State, federal and accrediting bodies set standards that outline characteristics networks must have to be sufficiently robust. While these standards vary, they all aim to ensure the network contains enough providers to adequately provide members access to care within acceptable time and distance requirements.

Negotiating Network Contracts

Ultimately, your ability to develop and manage your network will depend on the contracts you design and implement with your providers. These contracts can be very complex, and they need to define everything from workflow and performance expectations to provider incentives and reporting requirements (see Figure 6.5).

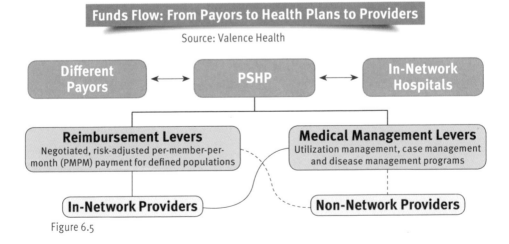

Funds Flow: From Payors to Health Plans to Providers

Source: Valence Health

Different Payors ↔ **PSHP** ↔ **In-Network Hospitals**

Reimbursement Levers
Negotiated, risk-adjusted per-member-per-month (PMPM) payment for defined populations

Medical Management Levers
Utilization management, case management and disease management programs

In-Network Providers **Non-Network Providers**

Figure 6.5

These services and features should be designed to reinforce your PSHP's value-based care arrangements, further differentiating your PSHP from traditional health plans. Network contracting has a big impact on whether you will be able to work within your premium rates or not. If you end up paying your contracted providers too much or you do not have enough control over their outcomes and costs, you will end up giving away much of the profit you should have made on those rates.

Therefore, it is incredibly important to thoughtfully gather a team who will create these contracts in a way that makes all parties involved come away happy. Frequently, this involves bringing together your health plan representatives and care delivery leadership when conducting contract negotiations with prospective providers and facilities. This can reinforce your organization's payor-provider alignment and further articulate your value proposition. It also helps provide immediate answers about your entire organization, which can facilitate a successful, timely contracting process.

Your team must also be sensitive to and mindful of contracts that providers and facilities have with other payors. Some providers may not want to disrupt the payor relationships they currently have, while others may be seeking a more rewarding partnership. This dynamic often depends upon your local area's payor mix and each payor's reputation.

Expert Insight

"In provider contracting, some health plans may feel that they are at a disadvantage in negotiating, so the temptation is to enter into complicated contracts just because the health plan feels that the leverage is on the other side and a big hospital system may ask for some concessions. But there is a downstream effect to every concession the health plan makes.

Having a knowledgeable person — someone who understands the costs, terms of the agreement and administrative burden — is a core competency for any new PSHP that is holding contract negotiations. That is why some clients partner with Valence Health, especially if they are going through a contract negotiation. They can ask us questions and we can give them guidance."

– Anthony Gutierrez
Vice President of Operations, Valence Health

Similarly, if you want to contract with a hospital that is part of a larger health system, you may be required to contract with all of that system's hospitals to gain access. This may prevent contract negotiations, or it is possible this health system will fulfill your network adequacy requirements without driving substantial utilization away from your affiliated healthcare organization (see the *Evaluating Contracts with Entire Health Systems* case study for more information).

Case Study:
Evaluating Contracts with Entire Health Systems – *Dean Health Plan*

"There are times during network development when a PSHP may identify a hospital located in their core service area that would be instrumental in achieving network adequacy, but competes with its sponsoring health system. However, sometimes these hospitals are part of a broader health system that demands a contract with their entire system in order for your members to utilize the one hospital needed for your network. At Dean Health Plan, we have dealt with this exact issue.

Sometimes this can simply be an insurmountable barrier, but other times, network balance may be achieved. In some cases, contracting with a particular health system will cause your affiliated healthcare organization to lose too many patients to competing facilities in the area, undermining your health system's strategy. In this scenario, this contract may not be a viable option, and your health plan will need to find other ways to fill the network gaps or focus on other geographies.

On the other hand, if the geographical footprint of the other health system and your sponsoring healthcare organization overlap very little, then this contract may be a viable option to consider. The other organization's facilities may be distant from your core service area and target market, so the fact that the other hospitals are included in your network becomes manageable. If it does not overly disrupt your affiliated healthcare organization's proportion of services and the medical costs of the other system are competitive, then this may be a promising solution to your network gap and could even create the foundation for potential care delivery collaboration in the future. Although some of the membership served becomes more of a 'pure insurance play,' it can be an important part of the overall balancing act for a PSHP's network and the overall strategy of its sponsoring system."

– J.C. McWilliams
System Vice President of Managed Care and Network Management, Dean Health Plan

There are three main different types of contracts your PSHP can use: proprietary contracts for local in-network providers, wrap network contracts for distant in-network providers and single-case agreement contracts for out-of-network providers.

- **Proprietary Contracts**

  Proprietary, or direct, contracts are used to partner with physicians or facilities to fulfill your plan's network adequacy requirements. In addition to physicians in your affiliated healthcare organization, your PSHP may need to fill in its network gaps by forming proprietary contracts with outside providers and facilities, depending on the size of your affiliated healthcare organization's geographic footprint and the breadth and depth of its services. These contracts allow your PSHP to offer services across a broader geographic area or facilitate referrals to tertiary care, quaternary care or specialty services that are not available through your core network.

- **Wrap Contracts**

  Wrap networks provide access to in-network providers, hospitals and ancillary services throughout the nation, providing a broad network for when your members are out of area and require medical care. Most PSHPs form a single contract with a national preferred provider organization (PPO) network to form a wrap network. Plan members can identify the wrap network from their ID card and hopefully access the closest in-network provider.

- **Single-Case Contracts**

  Not all members can locate their wrap network, especially in emergency situations, and some may receive services from out-of-network providers. To avoid paying full charges on one of these claims, the PSHP will generally attempt to contract with the out-of-network provider to establish a list of allowed charges, or discounted fees, that reduce the cost of medical services. If the provider accepts the contract, the discount will be applied to re-price the claim. However, if this cannot occur, your PSHP can attempt to form a single-case agreement with the provider to see if a discount can be secured for the specific claim.

The timeline for establishing these contracts will vary significantly depending on the complexity of the product and the provider's previous relationship with your health plan or its affiliated healthcare organizations. Initially, the process of creating a proprietary contract with a new provider may take nine to 18 months. However, once a relationship is established, this process will likely gain momentum, allowing new products to be added faster.

If your health plan or the contracted entity wants to change or reopen the contracted agreement, there are several ways this can be initiated. Frequently, this will occur at the time the contract would otherwise auto-renew. By following the notice requirements in the contract, either party can formally request contract renegotiations rather than automatic renewal.

If the contract needs to be renegotiated prior to the renewal, this can occur at any time by simply following the notice requirements. Other contracts are designed to contain specific triggers that will automatically reopen the contract. These triggers are customizable, but frequently occur when a certain level of membership, volume or quality is reached.

Orchestrating Network Reimbursement

Traditionally, providers view insurers as little more than a used car/bus salesman who stands in the way of getting a good deal and does not care about his customers. To some degree, insurers are a middle man; they receive premiums from members and pay a percentage to providers for care rendered, yet offer very limited or no care provision themselves. Insurers also can draw out the reimbursement process for providers, much like that used car salesman who frequently leaves you sitting in his office to "talk with the boss."

When a PSHP is the insurer, providers that contract with you are much less likely to feel antagonized. Let's face it: providers and insurers are one and the same in a PSHP, and this is something that should be made clear to all involved when you are working out compensation rates and packages with other providers. Since doctors like to be paid quickly for appropriately delivered healthcare, any speed bumps related to reimbursement will likely throw a monkey wrench into the engine of your PSHP. Setting clear guidelines and expectations for reimbursement right from the start will help greatly, as everyone will be on the same page and providers will know when and how they can expect to be paid (see the *Understanding Premium Price* case study for more information).

Case Study
Understanding Premium Price – *Land of Lincoln Health*

"To make our plans competitive, we decided to have transparent, open dialogues with our providers about what we are trying to accomplish. For us, that involved putting a blank piece of paper on the table and saying to the provider, 'If you tell us what you would like to get paid, we will model it for you and show you how that would translate into our products' premiums.'

When we came back, we lay down the actuarially validated numbers and say, 'This is how those rates translate into this month's premium price.' We then disclose in a very transparent conversation all the components that affect that monthly premium price, including plan design, the risk corridors and our utilization factors.

Then we ask them the hard question: 'If it stacks up this way in the marketplace, do you believe a consumer will buy this product?' It becomes a very enlightening discussion."

– Daniel Yunker
CEO, Land of Lincoln Health
President and CEO, Metropolitan Chicago Healthcare Council

Value-Based Reimbursement Options Your PSHP Can Use

As the bus driver, you get to align incentives across your network. Your plan also has a range of options to choose from — all of which will hopefully put your fellow network contractees in great clinical and financial control of the care they deliver (as shown in Figure 6.6).

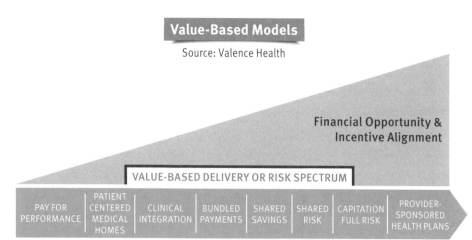

Figure 6.6

By working with providers to structure appropriate outcomes-focused, not volume-focused reimbursement models instead of focusing on rate negotiations, you will be able to have a much more open, transparent dialogue about your PSHP's population health objectives. In turn, other providers should be much more willing to work with you on how they are compensated.

While we know that your PSHP will have to use some amount of fee-for-service (FFS) reimbursement, our hope is that you will use your new payor status to help your larger provider community embrace value-based reimbursement through all of your contracting and reimbursement discussions.

To arm you for the conversations, we included a brief discussion on several of the most common value-based reimbursement models.

Pay for Performance

In the early 2000s, the concept of "pay for performance" (P4P) emerged as a popular tactic for aligning provider payment with value. Under the typical P4P model, financial incentives or disincentives are tied to measured performance. Simply stated, providers receive performance-based adjustments to their FFS rates, usually bonuses for exceeding standards in a particular metric and occasionally penalties for falling short. In most cases, the model requires the ability to establish clinical quality benchmarks, as well as to collect, measure and report results.

For example, a P4P immunization program could be set up where the goal for a pediatric practice is to immunize 80 percent of its patients by age 2, in accordance with the nationally accepted immunization guidelines. A provider that exceeds that goal would receive bonuses in addition to the standard FFS immunizations reimbursement rate from the payor.

The P4P model is not perfect. Often, the incentives are too small to change physician behavior or the patient population being affected is too small to institutionalize change. It also remains essentially a FFS model with respect to "rewards," with providers receiving higher payments in return for rendering more service.

Bundled Payment/Episode of Care

As its name suggests, the bundled payment/episode-of-care model provides a single negotiated payment for all services related to a specified procedure or condition, such as pregnancy or knee replacement surgery. The model bases provider payment amounts on the costs of adhering to clinical standards of care, risk stratification and complication allowances. It can also incentivize provider performance based on a comprehensive scorecard.

Under an episode-of-care payment system, providers automatically benefit from any savings they generate by improving efficiency within episodes. Under a comprehensive-care payment system, providers also can benefit from the savings they achieve by preventing unnecessary episodes of care. The payor, meanwhile, saves money by paying a provider less money per episode than it has in the past. Moreover, the payor knows upfront how much it will be spending, rather than having to wait to see whether any savings will be achieved.

Under a CMS bundled-payment model being piloted at a handful of hospitals, a single discounted payment is provided to the hospitals and physicians for an episode of care, such as a surgical or medical diagnosis-related group (DRG). In turn, the hospitals may pay physicians up to 125 percent of Medicare FFS rates and share up to 50 percent of savings with Medicare patients.

One financial downside for providers associated with this model is having to cover the costs of services for such procedures or conditions that exceed the agreed-upon reimbursement amount. Another drawback is that providers are ultimately forced to treat more episodes to increase their income; this can make bundled payment arrangements a more sophisticated form of FFS.

Shared Savings (One-Sided Risk)

Shared-savings arrangements represent a potentially higher level of reward by compensating providers who reduce total healthcare spending on their patients below an expected level set by the payor. The provider is then entitled to get a portion or share of the savings. The idea is that the insurer spends less on a patient's treatment than it would have otherwise spent and the provider receives more revenue than it otherwise would have expected (see Figure 6.7).

Shared-Savings Payment Cycle

Source: Valence Health

Agreement	Billing & Claims	Analysis	Payout	Bonus Distribution
A relationship is struck between providers and payors including patient attribution, covered services and estimated medical costs.	Providers submit claims as they would under a fee-for-service structure — nothing new.	The payor and provider each review medical costs to see what, if any, savings were achieved.	Payor pays provider organization a bonus based on savings achieved.	Provider organization divides total bonus amount among program provider participants (e.g., hospital, specialists, primary care, etc.)

Figure 6.7

Under the Medicare Shared Savings Program (MSSP), integrated groups of providers earn bonuses for demonstrating slower spending growth for patient care relative to their peers. While the program has different tracks and very specific requirements, the basic principles of MSSP allow some amount of the savings to be kept by the provider organizations, with another portion of the savings returned to CMS.

Shared-savings programs, however, do suffer from several significant shortcomings. For one, they may not pay for some primary care services, such as nurse case managers for chronic disease patients, and phone and email consults with other physicians. In many cases, they also require upfront spending by the provider to implement processes or technology changes necessary to achieve success. While revenue may increase from such programs, it could be months or years in the future before performance improvement has been assessed and program investments have been recouped.

Also, providers with the highest rates of hospital admissions, highest use of unnecessary procedures and other resource wasters tend to benefit most under the shared-savings model. In contrast, the best performers — those with relatively low costs and high quality of care — already are "saving" Medicare and other payors significant amounts of money, but do not get any more rewards than resource wasters. Through the shared-savings model, the first group can improve relatively easily, thus becoming eligible for a large reward, while the second may need to invest significantly more resources to obtain the rewards.

Finally, shared-savings programs ultimately may prove unsustainable. Even if healthcare delivery costs remain lower than they would otherwise have been expected to remain, critics say payors will find it difficult to continue making shared-savings payments indefinitely based on savings achieved in the past, particularly as the providers and their patients change over time. This may deter providers from making large investments in care improvements that would need to be paid off over a multiyear period.

Shared Risk

Shared risk models could be described as the "next level" of risk arrangements, under which providers receive performance-based incentives to share cost savings, combined with disincentives to share the excess costs of healthcare delivery.

Shared Risk with Corridors Arrangement

Source: Valence Health

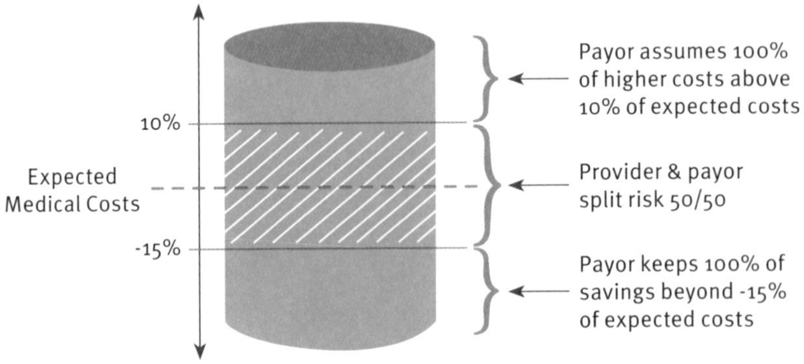

10%

Expected
Medical Costs

-15%

Payor assumes 100%
of higher costs above
10% of expected costs

Provider & payor
split risk 50/50

Payor keeps 100% of
savings beyond -15%
of expected costs

Figure 6.8

This model is based on an agreed-upon budget with a payor, and calls for the provider to cover a portion of costs if savings targets are not achieved; this portion could be a percentage of the premium (e.g., 30 percent of the overall premium flows to provider) or a set amount (e.g., 50/50 sharing of excess costs). As expected under this model, providers take on more risk for both achieving savings and failing to achieve savings, which is known as upside and downside risk (see Figure 6.8). At Valence Health, shared risk arrangements are the point at which we say you are moving from risk "lite" to real risk assumption for the care you deliver.

However, this model requires that payors are willing to structure a shared-risk program that meets the needs and capabilities of the provider organization. If the payor is interested in passing along more risk to the provider than that organization is willing to accept, the provider organization can look to third parties to offer what is referred to as stop-loss insurance to cover costs that exceed a specified amount. In such arrangements, the provider organization pays a fixed fee for that third-party insurer to accept all the financial risk beyond a certain level.

An alternate method of limiting risk is including risk-corridor arrangements (again, see Figure 6.8). Corridors protect from high losses, but also obstruct opportunities for large gains (for more information on risk corridors, refer to Chapter 10, "Actuarial Considerations and Financial Management"). All of these risk-limiting strategies increase the likelihood that the payor and the provider organization can reach an agreement.

Full Risk: Capitation Models

Under a capitated-payment model, a provider organization, or group of organizations, receive from the payor a set payment per patient for specified medical services. In this way, the provider takes on 100 percent of the insurance risk for the covered patient and services. These payments are usually in the form of a monthly per-patient fee. These fees are determined by actuarial analysis of historic costs of the patient population to be covered by the capitated model. These fees are adjusted to reflect the "acuity" or "level of risk" associated with the patient population. Then, the provider organization or group of organizations must determine how to divide up the single capitated payment. More often than not, this funds disbursement is done using a combination of incentives and FFS agreements.

There are two basic capitation models: "global" or "full capitation" and "partial" or "blended capitation":

- Global capitation describes an arrangement where a provider organization, or group of organizations, come together to receive a single fixed payment for the entirety of healthcare services a patient (or "member" in the eyes of the payor) could receive. This includes primary care, hospitalizations, specialist care and ancillary services.

- Partial capitation is where the single monthly fee that is paid to the provider only covers a defined set of healthcare services. Services not covered usually are still paid for on an FFS basis. For example, it is not uncommon to see a partial capitation model that only includes physician services (primary care and specialty) and laboratory services, but excludes hospital-based care, pharmacy and mental health benefits.

Regardless of whether the capitation is global or partial, the provider is at full risk for the services that are covered. This means that providers reap the rewards of providing care at a cost below the capitated rate, but also bear the risk if the cost of care exceeds the capitated amounts. As with other forms of risk, providers can employ stop-loss insurance to limit the upper-end of their exposure.

Maintaining an Established Network

After you have made strides in developing your network and negotiating contracts and reimbursement models, you will need to keep an eye on the management of your network, just as you always keep an eye on your mirrors when you drive your PSHP "bus." Networks can change as quickly as the road before you. Your member populations may shrink or grow and their needs will change over time, so you need to be able to adapt quickly if you want to be successful.

Communicate Effectively

One of the best ways to maintain your network is to make sure your providers are kept up-to-date. It is very important to keep your providers aware of any changes that may come as a result of your managing the PSHP's dynamic network. Just as you would tell your mechanic about anything new that has happened with your bus when you bring it in for an oil change, your providers need to know any important information that may affect them as your network grows or shifts. They cannot do their jobs without all of the facts.

Eliminate Underperforming Providers

Another logical practice after you have developed a stable network of providers is to work to retain your high-quality providers, while eliminating the lower-quality ones from your network. If your reimbursement model ties performance measures to provider reimbursement, then the pocketbooks of your lower-quality providers may do this task for you.

Otherwise, data becomes crucial; it is like the computer in your bus. It monitors everything that is going on, and lets you know which pieces are working correctly and which are underperforming. Data is vital for any conversation you may have with underperforming providers to either help them improve or transition them out of your network. It also provides you with performance baselines for providers that you can compare against any backdrop, be it local or nationwide.

Providers know what these baselines are for the care that they deliver — they know what makes care ideal or poor, and they know which providers are deemed high quality and which are low quality based on their history or "mileage." Performance data allows you to clearly see how each of your providers is impacting your network.

> **Expert Insight**
>
> *"We are embarking on a time when data and connectivity are starting to evolve in the healthcare industry with the help of the healthcare information exchanges and the regional sharing of clinical data.*
>
> *Over a period of time, it will become pretty clear which providers are performing or not performing in this value equation. Many of the disparities we have discussed over the years — sicker patients, varying quality of care and so forth — will all start to normalize because of big data."*
>
> **– Daniel Yunker**
> CEO, Land of Lincoln Health
> President and CEO, Metropolitan Chicago Healthcare Council

However, you also must look beyond the data, and understand the demographics and the challenges your hospitals and providers face in caring for your members. Many providers believe the members they serve are truly different and that the work that they do is unique and hard to quantify.

If you fail to understand their challenges, the providers will think that you do not understand their perspective and are not willing to work with them. This is where having a physician as a part of your management staff can be vital — providers are going to be much more skeptical of and resistant to a PSHP administrator talking to them about treatment habits and performance data, even if the administrator has the data in hand. Physicians are much more likely to be responsive to an administrator who happens to be a clinician because they trust someone who knows what it is like to be in the trenches with them.

Identify Network Leakage

Regardless of how hard you have worked in developing and maintaining your provider network, there will be a number of your members who, for one reason or another, seek care outside of your network. Maybe one went to an out-of-network specialist based on a word-of-mouth referral from a coworker. Or another broke his leg while waterskiing on vacation and simply went to the nearest emergency department in the area.

"Leakage," where members seek care outside of the network through referrals or by their own choice, can significantly impact your PSHP's ability to be efficient and profitable. Whether through referrals or not, leakage is a two-tire blowout on the bus that is your PSHP; not only are you losing money through not providing care (which may be going to a competitor), but you are also losing in terms of your organization's reputation. Members would not seek care outside of the network if they truly thought your network provided the best care or access available to them.

Actionable Strategies for Preventing Network Leakage
Source: Valence Health

✓ **Build patient engagement into your value proposition**
- Establish a proven reputation for patient care
- Enhance your network's unique value as a collaborative care unit
- Make your patients want to stay in network

✓ **Use data to locate plan levers**
- Identify areas of physician improvement
- Monitor population health needs and corresponding medical management programs
- Collaborate with non-traditional providers to improve access, quality and cost

✓ **Enhance transparent physician communication**
- Give physicians a voice in designing network management
- Clearly communicate who is in network
- Connect with your physicians through multiple channels (one-on-ones, forums, webinars, email, committee, etc.)

✓ **Create incentive models to reward in-network physicians**
- Set quality metric and performance level goals
- Recognize physicians for forward-thinking work
- Appropriately reward in-network referrals

✓ **Form a positive, trusting relationship with patients**
- Develop effective patient collateral
- Provide deep, consistent patient engagement and education
- Discuss the purpose of new initiates that aim to improve the patient experience

Figure 6.9

The good news is that patient leakage can be minimized (see Figure 6.9 for actionable strategies). While some organizations believe that putting a greater focus on physician-hospital integration will lead to more referrals back to their hospitals, this really only addresses the symptoms of the problem, not the root cause. It is like if you noticed your bus was leaking oil and you brought it to your mechanic to have the oil topped off, rather than finding out why it was leaking in the first place.

Data and analytics will be your trusted mechanic, helping you understand where your patients are going when they leave your network and why. They will allow you to study your members' behavior across service lines, geographies and physicians – both inside and outside of your PSHP's network. You may discover that some of the leakage relates to things like geography or distance, reluctance to see a new provider, specialists of substandard quality or referrals to providers who are booked for long periods. These all are things that analysis and data can help you identify and address (see the *Mitigating Patient Leakage* case study for more information). ⊘

Case Study:
Mitigating Patient Leakage – *Metropolitan Chicago Healthcare Council*

"In the past, providers typically didn't want to believe that their patients go to different places. But I will wholeheartedly tell you — since we at the Metropolitan Chicago Healthcare Council also run the metro-Chicago health information exchange — we know there are a lot of patients going to a lot of other places.

Some of it is for convenience: I may have a personal care physician, but if I have a sore throat, that doesn't mean I want to wait two weeks to see my physician. Instead, I will probably go to the immediate care and that immediate care might be in a totally different health system than the one my physician works for.

I think this will continue to evolve with the health information exchange. What the health information exchange creates is an informed, connected healthcare community with the ability to conduct analytics for its population, manage population health, clinically integrate the markets it serves and truly evaluate the question of how we are delivering value. In the end, that is the question that needs to be answered."

– Daniel Yunker
CEO, Land of Lincoln Health
President and CEO, Metropolitan Chicago Healthcare Council

Tracking Key Health Plan Network Development and Management Metrics

Performing regular data analysis can help your PSHP maximize its return on investment and identify both early warning signs of trouble and indicators of success. By tracking key inputs and outputs, you can continually enhance your health plan so it retains members, remains financially stable and earns high patient satisfaction scores. Below are key network development and management metrics that should be measured continuously:

- Plan's claim expense
- Network providers' patient satisfaction scores
- Number and type of network gaps
- Network's level of access
- Network providers' business hours
- Publicly available quality information
- Fulfillment of credentialing standards
- Fulfillment of network adequacy standards
- Fulfillment of regulations and accreditation requirements
- Number and type of provider incentives
- Contract timelines and key requirements
- Provider reimbursement cycle time
- Network providers' performance data
- Member physician attribution changes
- Members' demographics (name, date of birth, gender, etc.)
- Members' medical conditions (diabetes, arthritis, high blood pressure, etc.)
- Patient leakage rate

Industry Terminology Related to Network Development and Management

Complication Allowance   When using bundled payments for reimbursement, some contracts include an ability to distinguish routine costs of care from costs associated with complications. These complications can become part of a warranty allowance that is built into each bundled payment and thus creates a margin opportunity for the participating providers.

Source: Health Care Incentives Improvement Institute

Medical Diagnosis-Related Group   Under Medicare's inpatient prospective payment system, each case is categorized into a diagnosis-related group (DRG), which has a payment weight assigned to it based on the average resources used to treat Medicare patients in that group.

Source: CMS.gov

Quaternary Care   Very specialized and highly unusual care that is not offered in every hospital or medical setting, e.g., experimental medicine and procedures or highly uncommon, specialized surgeries.

Source: Patients.About.com

Risk Stratification   A systematic process for identifying and predicting patient risk levels relating to healthcare needs, services and coordination. It involves use of algorithms and registries, payor data, physician/provider judgment/input and patient self-assessments and experiences.

Source: New Jersey Academy of Family Physicians

Stop-Loss Premium   The dollar amount of claims filed for eligible expenses at which point you have paid 100% of your out-of-pocket and the insurance begins to pay at 100%. Stop-loss is reached when an insured individual has paid the deductible and reached the out-of-pocket maximum amount of coinsurance.

Source: Healthinsurance.org

Value-Based Care   Linking provider payments to improved performance by healthcare providers. This form of payment holds healthcare providers accountable for both the cost and quality of care they provide. It attempts to reduce inappropriate care and to identify and reward the best-performing providers.

Source: HealthCare.gov

Chapter Seven
Medical Management

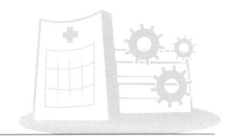

The healthcare industry is moving from a "more you charge, the more you get paid" mindset to a value-based way of providing healthcare (volume to value). This change is starting to bend the cost curve, which is why it is important for your provider-sponsored health plan (PSHP) and its affiliated health systems, hospitals and physicians to be aligned. All healthcare professionals know that an inpatient admission is not always an ideal health outcome. As health plan administrators, you will become even more acutely aware that your plan's clinical and financial mission is to keep patients healthy and out of the hospital.

As a PSHP, one of the most critical functions you will rely on to achieve this mission – essentially keeping your bus safely on the road – is medical management (see Figure 7.1). In effect, these services become your PSHP's steering wheel, directing suitable information and resources to all of your members in an effort to engage them and make them take a more active role in their healthcare.

Medical Management's Three Critical Components

Source: Valence Health

Utilization Management (UM)	The evaluation of the medical necessity, appropriateness and efficiency of the use of healthcare services, procedures and facilities under the provisions of the applicable health benefits plan, sometimes called "utilization review."
Case Management (CM)	A collaborative process that helps consumers manage their comprehensive health needs through communication and available resources to promote quality, cost-effective outcomes. A health professional case manager assesses, plans, implements, coordinates, monitors and evaluates options for consumers, their families, caregivers and the healthcare team (including providers) to promote these outcomes.
Disease Management (DM)	The processes and people concerned with improving or maintaining health in large populations. It is concerned with common chronic illnesses or conditions and the reduction of future complications associated with those diseases.

Figure 7.1

Your plan also will need medical management to become accredited by the National Committee for Quality Assurance (NCQA) or Utilization Review Accreditation Commission (URAC). While these accreditations are not mandatory if you only offer Medicare and Medicaid plans, they are required for public exchange participation (see Figure 7.2). They also are seen as the health insurance industry's seal of approval and are credentials that most of your competitors will likely have (for more information on accreditation, refer to Chapter 11, "Compliance").

> **Expert Insight**
>
> *"NCQA accreditation is important if you want to get into the health plan business. It is critical to have an external review system that when completed, says a health plan meets all of the industry's requirements."*
>
> **– Sue Price, RN, MS**
> Director of Medical Management, Valence Health

There are several other medical management requirements that are mandatory. The Centers for Medicare & Medicaid Services (CMS) and state Medicaid programs have required standards for services in case management (CM) and disease management (DM) that your organization must follow if your PSHP decides to offer plans to those payors. On top of that, states can have their own unique requirements beyond those associated with federal Medicaid requirements.

For example, if a large portion of the state's population is at risk for diabetes, then your state Medicaid agency may require your organization to provide diabetes medical management programs. Regardless of the exact circumstances, you need to know the specific requirements that apply to your health plan and set aside resources to fulfill them. Failing to do so could lead to minor and severe consequences, ranging from corrective action plans and fines to loss of your licensure or termination of your health plan (for more information on these and other consequences, refer to Chapter 11, "Compliance").

Above and beyond these requirements, your health plan and all of its affiliated provider organizations have the responsibility to decide how best to provide medical management services and to continuously reevaluate these decisions over time. As a health plan, in conjunction with your network providers, you have the ability and responsibility to improve patient health. Regardless of whichever execution strategy your PSHP selects, meaning whether you choose to build, buy or partner/outsource all or some portion of your medical management functions, what ultimately matters is that everyone works together to attain the common goal of providing members with the best care possible at the lowest possible costs. Just remember that executing any type of a change in your plan's utilization management (UM), CM or DM executional strategy will take time.

National Recognition of NCQA and URAC Accreditation

NCQA and URAC are two nationally recognized accrediting entities that allow health plans to validate their level of quality and accountability. This can help distinguish notable health plans from the competition and satisfy customer's demands for value, performance and transparency. Multiple states across the nation recognize NCQA and/or URAC accreditation:

States Recognizing NCQA Accreditation
Source: NCQA

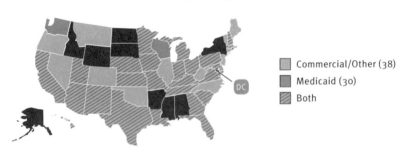

42 states recognize NCQA health plan accreditation in whole or part in either their commercial market and/or their Medicaid managed care programs.

Government Recognition of URAC Accreditation
Source: URAC

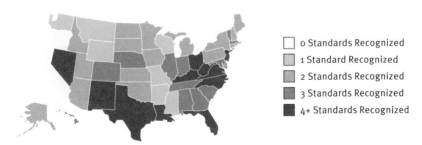

48 states and the District of Columbia recognize individual URAC accreditation standards.

Figure 7.2

Utilization Management (UM)

UM is the most traditional component of medical management and will offer your PSHP a system of checks and balances. UM's job is to ensure members get the right care at the right time in the right place. However, successful PSHPs often reduce or eliminate the need for traditional UM processes by facilitating close collaboration between healthcare providers and their health plan.

> **Expert Insight**
>
> *"To successfully perform medical management, good physician leadership and involvement is key. When you can make the entire care team — nurses, office staff, etc. — part of medical management design work, that's always optimal.*
>
> *As a health plan, you will have to help providers change their way of doing things, like admitting a knee-replacement patient to home health services rather than to an inpatient rehab after surgery when appropriate. If you really want to cement those kinds of changes, care team involvement is essential and will help assure that your network's providers are really aligned with new value-based care protocols and delivery models."*
>
> **– Lori Fox Ward, RN, BSN**
> Senior Vice President of Market Solutions, Valence Health

At PSHPs more so than at traditional plans, there is a prime opportunity to form an integrated leadership team that regularly solicits nurse and physician input into your plan's UM rules design process. In fact, some of Valence Health's PSHP clients reduce or eliminate the need for some forms of UM because the plan's physicians and nurses agree to follow evidence-based practices and make effective decisions on the front end (see Figure 7.3 for the three forms of UM). By having your plan's physician leaders tell other physicians about new UM protocols, your plan will likely enjoy greater physician buy-in and adherence to the rules.

Additionally, UM reviews allow health plans to monitor and control service delivery. The UM rules your plan has defined are typically for services that the industry continuously identifies as high-cost, easily overused or potentially cosmetic in nature, which would require review on an individual basis. When these services are prescribed by a physician, the information will be reviewed by your PSHP to ensure the service request meets established nationally recognized criteria.

Utilization Management Types and Timing Relative to Care Delivery

Source: Valence Health

Prospective Review	Precertification that occurs prior to medical services being delivered
Concurrent Review	Verification of medical necessity that occurs while in the hospital, between admission and discharge
Retrospective Review	Review of the delivered services that occurs after the date of service

Figure 7.3

These UM checks and balances, regardless of how your organization specifically executes them, can lead to substantial benefits for both the health plan and its provider network. Not only can it lower claim expenses by preventing unnecessary services, duplicative care and overutilization, but it also can function as a guiding mechanism for patient and provider behavior.

If physicians have access to current evidence-based practices and have incentives to use them, then this can guide their decisions toward delivering the best quality care, especially in contrast to the fee-for-service model that has no rewards or penalties. Likewise, both patients and providers tend to think twice or try another technique before pursuing services that require prior authorization. These techniques also can help prevent unnecessary services like prescribing an MRI for a patient who has a headache, but no neurological problems. It also can work as a filter to help identify physicians who are consistently prescribing services that go against your PSHP's guidelines.

However, it is not only your physician representatives and your plan's executive staff who are calling the shots. You also need to ensure any rules and UM activities comply with state and federal regulations, which are designed to protect all patients and will vary by state. As a PSHP, you also can help your provider and patient community to understand when there are new rules or regulations impacting your plan's UM policies and procedures, which will help everyone adhere to these new or revised guidelines.

A common requirement for proving UM compliance is obtaining a Utilization Review Agents (URA) license. Applying for this license involves submitting an application to your local department of insurance that describes your PSHP's UM program and how your plan conducts UM activities (for more information on URA licenses, refer to Chapter 11, "Compliance").

Profile:
Health Plan Utilization Management Nurse

Utilization Management Nurses (UMN) are responsible for executing utilization review functions to ensure high-quality, cost-effective medical outcomes. By discussing clinical information and plan requirements with appropriate healthcare providers and members, the UMN meets patient care needs, while optimizing member benefits. These nurses also:

- Maintain the appropriate levels of care and cost-effective medical outcomes by assessing the medical necessity of precertification requests, concurrent reviews and retrospective reviews

- Verify the treatment's compliance with applicable criteria, medical policy, and the patients' insurance eligibility, benefits and contracts

- Help reduce length of stay and prevent hospitalizations when possible and appropriate

- Monitor utilization trends so that members can be referred to case management and disease management as needed

Common Qualifications:

- Bachelor's degree or associate's degree in nursing

- State licensure as a registered nurse (RN)

Desired Knowledge:

- Benefits, reimbursement and limitations of commercial, Medicare and/or Medicaid coverage

- Patient care, medical treatments, hospital procedures and medical management processes

- Utilization review process used by third-party insurers

Source: Valence Health

Case Management (CM)

While UM helps patients by ensuring they are getting the right services, case management (CM) does this on a much more personal level. Case managers and their care teams communicate directly with members and their families to respond to their individual needs. For example, say some members are auto-assigned to your Medicaid health plan by the state Medicaid agency. They are guaranteed Medicaid eligibility, but your health plan is responsible for understanding their health history, stratifying their healthcare risks, and providing medical management and care coordination (refer to Chapter 10, "Actuarial Considerations and Financial Management," for more details around risk stratification).

Your PSHP's case managers can effectively engage with your plan's members to both gather their health histories and educate these members by helping them navigate the healthcare and social service systems they may need to use. Case managers also can encourage your plan's members to complete a health risk assessment (HRA) or offer to complete it on members' behalf (for more information on HRAs, refer to Chapter 10, "Actuarial Considerations and Financial Management"). Additionally, case managers could help members arrange transportation to get to their doctor's appointment, transition them from out-of-network to in-network providers, or coach them on when to use their primary care physician rather than the emergency department (ED).

Regardless of the specific task, the goal of CM is to assist members individually by ensuring they stay healthy and are in the right care settings, receiving the right care when needed. This, in turn, should reduce the number of complications, hospitalizations, overall length of stay and ultimately, unnecessary healthcare services and claims (see Figure 7.4).

These diverse CM functions are divided into two main types: general case management and complex case management. As their names suggest, general case management provides services for more acute, short-term needs. This includes everything from coordinating services and driving initiatives in ED diversion programs to making follow-up phone calls with members after hospitalizations or ED visits. Complex case management focuses on cases with complex medical, behavioral and psychosocial needs that require longer-term, team-based assessments and care planning.

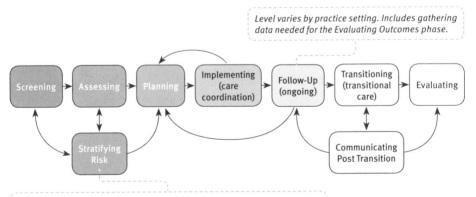

High-Level Case Management Process

Source: The Commission for Case Manager Certification's Case Management Body of Knowledge®

Figure 7.4

Profile:
Health Plan Case Manager

Case managers typically are responsible for the coordination and efficient use of healthcare resources for the provision of quality care for all patients assigned to them throughout the continuum of care. Case managers also:

* Assess and identify the patient's physical and psychosocial needs, and determine the appropriate healthcare services and level of care based on established benefits, protocols, pathways and evidence-based medicine tools

* Ensure appropriate levels of care by communicating with treating physicians and all other members of the healthcare team

* Identify other non-health community resources that could help the member

* Act as a member advocate by expediting and coordinating member care processes through the continuum, and working in concert with the healthcare delivery team to maintain high quality and cost-effective care

Common Qualifications:

* Bachelor degree in social work, public health or health education

* Certification in case management, health education or related fields

* Licensed Master Social Worker (LMSW) or Licensed Clinical Social Worker (LCSW)

Knowledge:

* Payor-specific case management guidelines

* Data-driven decision-making tools and their use

* Various reimbursement mechanisms, including third-party requirements

* Case management standards of practice that are in accordance with Case Management Society of America

Source: Valence Heath

In a health plan, these case management tasks generally are initiated by new data or a referral. For example, claims data may alert your plan administrators of members who have high costs, or HRA data may identify clients with high risks, like heavy tobacco use. Similarly, members may be selected for case management services via referrals from providers, community services or even UMN, who analyze and flag specific diagnoses, service accessed and admission patterns.

All of this information can help continuously identify trends that should be addressed by medical management programs. Once the member has been admitted to case management, these services and the corresponding care plans are communicated directly to the member's primary care physician.

> **Expert Insight**
>
> *"The most successful CM programs are the ones that are supported by the member's doctor. It is much more effective if the case manager can call the member and say, 'I am working with your physician and am here to help you learn about your diabetes.' In contrast, it can feel a lot like Big Brother is watching if the call comes and the person says, 'I'm from your health insurance company and I'd like to help you with your diabetes.'*
>
> *Patients most likely have a good relationship with their physician, so if a case manager can come in as an extension of that physician, then they can usually have a much more significant impact on helping the member get to an optimal state of well-being."*
>
> **– Sue Price, RN, MS**
> Director of Medical Management, Valence Health

In your PSHP, case managers may work for the hospitals in your network, your health plan, an outside partner or all three. Regardless, the important point is that all of the case managers work together to ensure members receive the appropriate help along and across their continuum of care (see the Health Plan Case Manager Profile sidebar). Now that you are driving the bus, your health plan will have to determine which CM resources are in the best position to provide CM services, and then offer them.

Disease Management (DM)

Along with offering personalized care through case management, your organization also will likely want to provide population-based services that provide education, information and care to groups of members who have a common disease or condition. This type of care is typically called disease management (DM).

DM focuses on managing conditions or a single disease to help patients better manage, stop or slow progression, improve their health and avoid future expenses. The goal is to help patients better understand the condition and its comorbidities so they can more effectively manage their health. To make your PSHP's DM impactful, you will want to conduct research to identify which diseases in your member population should be or could be better managed. Next, assessments must be conducted to truly determine how the specific condition is affecting your plan's members, where the members are in terms of controlling their disease or conditions, and what members might need to better manage the diseases.

This information, along with paid health plan claims, pharmacy information, lab results and electronic medical record data — when pulled together — can help your plan determine each member's level of risk. Once the at-risk patients are identified and stratified, your PSHP will want to decide what types of information it will want to push to members who have these conditions.

If you are offering DM to your members, your plan will need to access a library of educational materials. As discussed more extensively in Chapter 3, "Determining Your PSHP's Comprehensive Execution Strategy," you can build, buy or partner/outsource to set-up and maintain your DM resources. Your PSHP also will have to determine the types of interventions it will use — from mailings, over the phone or in-person meetings — and how your plan will go about stratifying your members' risk levels (see the case study, *Vendor Services for Disease Management*).

Case Study:
Vendor Services for Disease Management

"At Valence Health, we have programs for DM that are designed to meet NCQA accreditation requirements. We also use our population health technology and health plan business intelligence assets to aggregate our clients' health plan members' data so we can stratify the plan's population into three levels: well controlled, fairly controlled or poorly controlled. We also have developed a process for specific outreach depending on members' level of risk. Members in level one would get informational mailings, while level two members would get a mailing and a phone call with an assessment to obtain additional information.

For example, we could pull all of the members who are diagnosed with asthma and stratify them based on their claims and pharmacy data. In that case, members who have had an ED visit for their asthma are placed in level three, and may get a phone call to see if they'd like to join an asthma control group that meets monthly in their neighborhood and a home visit from a nurse. Those members with no recorded difficulty will be placed in level one and may only get a quarterly newsletter that contains asthma management tips."

– Sue Price, RN, MS
Director of Medical Management, Valence Health

After your initial DM processes are in place, and as more members join your plan, subsequent at-risk patients will be identified for disease management in many of the same ways that members are selected for case management, i.e., using HRA data and referrals from providers and UM.

Best-in-class health plan DM also assures that the primary care physicians of patients with "fairly controlled" or "poorly controlled" conditions are notified when their patients begin receiving DM services from the patient's health plan. However, providers of patients with "well controlled" conditions will simply be made aware of the DM services so they can recommend and share materials with patients on their specific conditions. In turn, when a patient's condition becomes more well controlled because of added interventions, the plan will also share this information with the patient's/member's physicians.

Profile:
Disease Management Specialists

Disease management specialists facilitate and perform outreach and telephonic assessments of populations with chronic diseases, like asthma and diabetes. DM activities can occur any time a member is enrolled in a health plan. Specialists also commonly:

- Assess and identify the patient's physical and psychosocial needs and determine the appropriate healthcare services and level of care based on established benefits, protocols, pathways and evidence-based medicine tools

- Select appropriate education materials and support for members with certain diseases or conditions

- Focus efforts on patient-centric education designed to optimize the member's health through proactive recognition of signs and symptoms, self-monitoring techniques, ongoing provider communication, the removal of barriers to care

- Act as a member advocate by expediting the care process through the continuum and working in concert with the healthcare delivery team to maintain high-quality and cost-effective care

Common Qualifications:

- Bachelor's or master's degree in health education, public health or health-related field

- Certified Health Education Specialist (CHES) or Master Certified Health Education Specialist (MCHES)

- Training in motivational interviewing

Knowledge:

- Health insurance criteria/guidelines

- Data-driven decision-making tools and their use

- Various criteria sets and reimbursement mechanisms, including third-party requirements

- Disease management standards of practice that are in accordance with payor-specific requirements/guidelines and other reputable associations and academic institutions

Source: Valence Heath

Some research has shown that DM does not always have a good return on investment (ROI) for reasons that include patients' mistrust of information provided by a health plan, difficulty reaching members and short timeframes often used by researchers to measure DM ROI. Therefore, the primary reason that many health plans offer DM is to fulfill regulations or accreditation requirements. As the driver of your PSHP's bus, this will be a decision that your leadership team will need to collectively make and own — knowing that DM provision is a must have if you are seeking accreditation.

Patient/Member Engagement

In the end, your organization's UM, CM and DM programs will be worthless if they cannot proactively communicate and build trust with members to effectively persuade them to start practicing healthy behaviors or stop making poor health choices (see Figure 7.5). Whether it is to take prescribed medication, start exercising or regularly visit their physician, your plan's UM, CM and DM programs' unified goal is to drive beneficial behaviors that will improve members' health and reduce expenses for the PSHP and its affiliated healthcare organization.

Patient Engagement – The Future Standard of Care

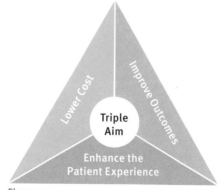

In today's healthcare environment, many organizations are setting their sights on the Triple Aim. This goal involves lowering costs, enhancing the patient experience, and improving outcomes. Organizations that fail to use patient engagement as an instrument for advancement may fall behind the future standards of care.

Figure 7.5

As this chapter mentioned earlier, with UM, CM and DM, your plan's patient/member engagement activities can be provided by your PSHP, the hospitals and other providers in your PSHP's network or by an outside partner. However you choose to implement these strategies, successful PSHPs most often treat patient engagement as a supporting strategy to your plan's UM, CM and DM efforts.

Studies have found that effective patient engagement not only has a positive impact on your patients, but on your organization as well. These organizational benefits include risk mitigation and improved quality, patient satisfaction, population health, improved healthcare economics and operational efficiency. However, to attain these benefits, there are a few useful things to know.

Patient/member engagement, regardless of who provides it, has changed dramatically over time. With the increase in data and personal electronic devices, an organization can no longer afford to use business models from a few decades ago. This traditional model is designed around episodic, acute events and provides retroactive, rather than proactive, engagement. In short, members are only engaged if they just had a medical procedure or have chronic, unmanaged conditions — not for preventive care.

As you take on this new role as a health insurer, your PSHP will need to think about how it can uniquely establish a meaningful relationship with its members to help them better manage their health. If your PSHP only has limited opportunities to engage, the chance of creating that bond lessens.

As Valence Health continues to work with PSHPs, we are encouraged by those that have abandoned old models of patient engagement and are leveraging technology to proactively reach out to their members (see the case study, *Engagement to Improve Patient Health*). In the traditional models, plans would send out mailers (which reached a high number of people, but were not very effective) or had their employees make phone calls (which were not scalable and very expensive).

Case Study:
Engagement to Improve Patient Health

"One PSHP sought to reach the segment of their population that was overdue for a mammogram and encourage them to schedule a screening. The organization identified 4,244 patients who were overdue for a mammogram, and then utilized our patient engagement call campaigns to explain the importance of the screening, as well as provide an opportunity to update their records or transfer directly to their provider to schedule.

In one month, it required 5,636 calls to connect with 24% of the population (1,016 patients). To replicate that outreach manually, it would have required an extensive amount of resources. By using our patient engagement platform, the PSHP was able to determine 14% of this population already had a mammogram. Therefore, their records needed to be updated and 11% of other patients were transferred to actually schedule. That was achieved in just one month, with no additional resources required from the organization."

– Devin Gross
CEO, Emmi Solutions

In the current technological age, there are better ways to reach members. There is texting, social media, and telephonic and web-based modes of communication that can be used strategically in facilitating your PSHP's engagement with patients. But before your organization can engage members, you need to know who they are and how to best connect with them. To do this effectively, this involves following the seven core competencies of patient engagement (see Figure 7.6).

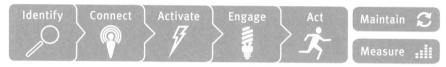

The Core Competencies of Patient Engagement

Source: Emmi Solutions

Identify | Connect | Activate | Engage | Act | Maintain | Measure

Identify: Identify patients and the messages they need to hear

Connect: Reach patients on their own terms, on the devices they prefer, in a language they understand

Activate: Inspire patients to care about their specific health issues

Engage: Give patients the tools and understanding needed for them to take their own action

Act: Encourage patients to take steps on their own to better manage their care

Maintain: Keep patients on the right path

Measure: Consistently measure outcomes at the individual level and in aggregate

Figure 7.6

Historically, health plans had no concept of targeting engagement based on an individual's personal preference, or demographic or psychosocial characteristics. However, these broader indicators can effectively change the content and medium through which a message is sent. Some people prefer to read, while others want to listen or watch.

Regardless, the point is that your members are going to have different preferences and your organization should respect these whenever possible. As the healthcare and insurance industry become more competitive, personalized engagement will become more prevalent. To start identifying preferences for member engagement, your PSHP will need data, because the more you know, the more you can target outreach initiatives.

There are three main types of data that will help your organization: claims data, clinical data and consumer data. The first two types are relatively standard and have been used for years to stratify patients into various levels of risk. The third one, however, is what organizations are just beginning to gather to help personalize their engagement. Consumer data includes demographic, psychosocial and self-reported data, or information on buying habits, FICO score, literacy level, etc. These data are gathered using surveys and tools, like the HRA and patient activation measures (see the case study, *Utilizing Data in Patient Engagement*).

Case Study:
Utilizing Data in Patient Engagement

"To effectively engage your members, it's important to attain information about them sooner rather than later. For example, if an individual is going to sign up on the exchanges, the first thing the health plan wants the person to do is complete a health risk assessment and then connect with a care coordinator. But engagement doesn't stop there. The plan needs to maintain a relationship with the member and continue to gather meaningful information that will help them better tailor the information to serve that person's unique needs.

Here's an example: The retail industry is very good at using customer relationship management systems. This is not prevalent in healthcare, but in my opinion, if a provider is going to start a health plan, then they need to think about their members the same way retailers think about their customers. To do that, they need to identify the systems that should be put in place and the best methods of gathering data so they can motivate individuals to do the things they want.

When you buy a product online, the company profiles you immediately and continues to gather more information about you over the years. Health plans need to think like this to effectively engage people — it is much more than just claims and clinical data."

– Devin Gross
CEO, Emmi Solutions

Now, some of your members will fill out these surveys or tools and consume your organization's engagement information regularly, especially if it provides the right information, at the right time through the right medium. But that certainly will not include everyone. You will soon discover that some members will not complete surveys or tools and will not consume your information. For those members, incentives can be an effective motivator.

Keep in mind that some states or types of plans prohibit or limit the use of incentives, so you will have to consult your local department of insurance, CMS and/or your state Medicaid agency if you are serving these payors to understand their boundaries. However, for those payors that allow it, incentives can effectively drive patient behavior. These incentives are often financial, like a gift card or lower premiums, but they can be anything — even a free car seat or athletic equipment — so long as it makes your members more likely to take the desired action. Whether it is fulfilling a wellness participation requirement, completing a shared decision-making program or attending all prenatal visits, these incentives can promote healthier behavior.

Case Study:
Incentivizing Physicians

"Health plans can effectively shape provider behavior through the use of physician incentives. One of our clients incentivized physicians by giving them control over patient involvement.

The plan articulated that the physicians would be held accountable for getting 30% of patients to participate in a shared decision-making program, but developing and deciding the process for doing so was entirely in the physicians' hands. As a result, the physicians developed an effective process and they met their goal that year."

– Devin Gross
CEO, Emmi Solutions

Incentives also can be directed toward physicians. This can start with simple things like submitting all claims electronically or putting protocols in place to improve Healthcare Effectiveness Data and Information Set (HEDIS) metrics. Whether it is your members or providers, incentives can help improve your population's health, initiate cost savings and improve quality. ⊘

Tracking Key Health Plan Medical Management Metrics

Performing regular data analysis can help your PSHP maximize its return on investment and identify both early warning signs of trouble and indicators of success. By tracking key inputs and outputs, you can continually enhance your health plan so it retains members, remains financially stable and earns high patient satisfaction scores. Below are key medical management metrics that should be measured continuously:

- Number of prior authorization requests
- Analysis of unnecessary services, duplicative care and overutilization
- Claim expenses
- Amount of inappropriate claims reimbursement
- Number of patients referred to and receiving care or disease management services
- Number of patients with high-risk scores and high costs
- Member demographics (name, date of birth, gender, etc.)
- Members' medical conditions (diabetes, arthritis, high blood pressure, etc.)
- Members' treatment information (medications, surgeries, physical therapy, etc.)

- Members' healthcare costs
- Number of patients referred to and receiving disease management services
- Organizational costs associated with chronic illnesses
- Percentage of members with well controlled, fairly controlled and poorly controlled diseases and conditions
- Changes in members' disease and condition controls status over time
- Overall length of stay
- Patient satisfaction scores
- Fulfillment of regulations and accreditation requirements
- Number and type of compliance violation consequences related to UM, CM and DM programs

Industry Terminology Related to Medical Management

Care Coordination   The deliberate organization of patient care activities between two or more participants (including the patient) involved in a patient's care to facilitate the appropriate delivery of healthcare services. Organizing care involves the marshalling of personnel and other resources needed to carry out all required patient care activities, and is often managed by the exchange of information among participants responsible for different aspects of care.

Source: Agency for Healthcare Research and Quality

Care Plan   A document that identifies healthcare orders for a patient and serves as a guide to care. It can either be written for an individual patient, be retrieved from a computer and individualized or be preprinted for a specific disease, condition or diagnosis and individualized to the specific patient. Standardized care plans are available for a number of patient conditions.

Source: "Miller-Keane Encyclopedia and Dictionary of Medicine, Nursing and Allied Health," Seventh Edition.

Case Management   A collaborative process that helps consumers manage their comprehensive health needs through communication and available resources to promote quality, cost-effective outcomes. A health professional case manager assesses, plans, implements, coordinates, monitors and evaluates options for consumers, their families, caregivers and the healthcare team, including providers, to promote these outcomes.

Source: Utilization Review Accreditation Commission

Comorbidity   The simultaneous presence of two chronic diseases or conditions in a patient.

Source: Merriam-Webster

Continuum of Care   A concept involving a system that guides and tracks patients over time through a comprehensive array of health services spanning all levels and intensity of care. The continuum of care covers the delivery of healthcare over a period of time, and may refer to care provided from birth to end of life. Healthcare services are provided for all levels and stages of care.

Source: Healthcare Information Management Systems Society

Disease Management   Refers to the processes and people concerned with improving or maintaining health in large populations. It is concerned with common chronic illnesses and the reduction of future complications associated with those diseases.

Source: Utilization Review Accreditation Commission

Evidence-Based Practices Applying the best available research results (evidence) when making decisions about healthcare. Healthcare professionals who perform evidence-based practice use research evidence along with clinical expertise and patient preferences.

Source: Effectivehealthcare.AHRQ.gov

Health Risk Assessment (HRA) A collection of health-related data that a provider can use to evaluate the health status and the health risk of an individual. The HRA will identify health behaviors and risk factors known only to the patient (e.g., physical activity and nutritional habits) for which the medical provider can provide tailored feedback in an approach to reduce the risk factors as well as the potential inevitability of the diseases to which they are related.

Source: CMS.gov

Healthcare Effectiveness Data and Information Set (HEDIS) A tool used by more than 90% of America's health plans to measure performance on important dimensions of care and service. Altogether, HEDIS consists of 81 measures across five domains of care. Because so many plans collect HEDIS data, and because the measures are so specifically defined, HEDIS makes it possible to compare the performance of health plans on an "apples-to-apples" basis.

Source: National Committee for Quality Assurance

Return on Investment (ROI) A performance measure used to evaluate the efficiency of an investment or to compare the efficiency of a number of different investments.

Source: Investopedia.com

Utilization Management (UM) The evaluation of the medical necessity, appropriateness and efficiency of the use of healthcare services, procedures and facilities under the provisions of the applicable health benefits plan, sometimes called "utilization review."

Source: Utilization Review Accreditation Commission

Utilization Review Agent (URA) People working on behalf of a health insurance company who review a request for medical treatment and confirm a health plan provides coverage for medical services. This helps the company minimize costs and determine if the recommended treatment is appropriate.

Source: Health.HowStuffWorks.com

Chapter Eight
Customer Service

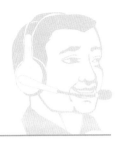

Every health plan strives to build loyalty and trust with its members, providers and payors. An integral part of both creating and maintaining those bonds will come from the types and level of customer service you provide to each of these key stakeholders. While customer service is not something new, having to deliver these services in the context of a health plan will likely create several new operational realities for your provider-sponsored health plan (PSHP).

First of all, health plan members and providers need prior approvals and benefits explanation questions answered — especially in the case of emergencies — 24 hours a day, seven days a week, every day of the year. Therefore, you will need a expertly trained customer service team, that is available both day and night, and is equally comfortable dealing with healthcare providers and members who may be highly frustrated.

Second, there will be times in your PSHP's regular business cycle when activities that generate customer service needs will both increase and decrease. For example, open enrollment season for any payor tends to create more questions and calls. There also may be local market issues, like a change in a state policy for Medicaid plans, which generate public awareness or press around health insurance and thereby generate more calls and questions from members and providers.

Third, your customer service team will have to be intimately familiar with the Health Insurance Portability and Accountability Act (HIPPA) protocols and any specific health insurance privacy laws that may be in play in your local market. Since health insurance is regulated at the state level, there may be additional requirements for both interactions and documentation of those interactions that your PSHP will have to meet and report on to your state Department of Insurance.

Fourth, you will have to make a strategic decision about whether your plan's customer service representatives (CSRs) will be reactive, proactive or both. Will they sit around waiting for the phone to ring or actively reach out to members who are entitled to a free flu shot during prime immunization season?

Case Study:
Proactive Customer Service

"You are probably aware that we experienced a mass casualty event just outside of Waco in West, Texas. We believe as many as 90 of our members might have been directly affected by this tragedy.

I was made aware that our Valence Health medical management team in Austin took the initiative to personally reach out to all 90+ members we show as maintaining residence in one of the affected zip codes. Information (or a voice message) was provided — outlining how the member may contact us for assistance with alternative access to care, replacement medications, etc.

This was not requested by the RightCare plan, but was instead taken on by the team in Austin as a simple means of ensuring we are doing everything we can to assist our members in this time of significant need."

– Dr. Scott Nicklebur
Chief Operating Officer/Chief Medical Officer, RightCare
Source: Internal Staff Memo

Customer service is a highly visible extension of your health plan and affiliated healthcare organization; as such, it needs to embody the same commitment to patient satisfaction and must focus on the member experience. As a PSHP, your organization is probably in a better position to fulfill this unified goal than traditional health plans due to the increased collaboration and alignment between your health plan and its provider network.

A customer service interaction should be a direct touch point with your PSHP's value proposition. Not only must the staff be professional and compassionate, but they also must be extremely knowledgeable and able to simply articulate the ins and outs of health insurance, and help your members and providers understand how the plan affects them. Therefore, your decision to build, buy or partner/outsource all or part of your plan's customer service capabilities will be a critically important executional strategy decision (refer to Chapter 3 for more about "Determining Your PSHP's Comprehensive Execution Strategy"). Also remember that once staff members are in place, they will have frequent training needs. Therefore, your executives also will need to decide how your PSHP will handle all ongoing customer service training.

To assure that you make this decision based on complete information, this chapter outlines some of the operational realities of having competitive customer service function and support. While many of your customer service operations' supportive technologies and metrics are uniform across industries, these standards maybe less familiar to some of the members of your PSHP's leadership team.

The Roles of a Customer Service Representative

When you buy a bus, you want one that is multi-functional and can fulfill all of your needs. Maybe you need one with enough seats for everyday purposes, a bathroom and luggage rack for passengers on long journeys and Wi-Fi and TVs for individuals who value their screen time. The bus must have all these features to work for you.

Just like your bus, CSRs must be able to serve multiple purposes; otherwise, they simply cannot do their job. During phone, email or online chat communications, these staff members must be everything from member or provider advocates to plan educators and sales representatives.

With their real-time access to both provider and member information systems, CSRs can view account details to perform a variety of tasks, which often are similar for providers and members (see Figure 8.1). For example, providers generally reach out to ensure they receive accurate reimbursement for their services, while members may want to know how much they need to pay.

Type of Customer Service Calls

Source: Valence Health

CSRs are responsible for assisting members, providers and brokers with a variety of questions and tasks. In general, the nature of these calls depend upon the caller's identity and frequently falls into the broad categories below:

	Eligibility	Claims	Commission	Benefits	Sales*	Contract
Member	✓	✓	∅	✓	✓	∅
Provider	✓	✓	∅	∅	∅	✓
Broker	∅	✓	✓	∅	✓	✓

To conduct sales activities, CSRs may need a sales licensure.

Figure 8.1

Additional tasks CSRs manage include:

- Updating demographic information and eligibility files, including adding or removing a dependent or providing a new address or phone number

- Relaying accurate and timely information regarding eligibility status and benefits information to confirm which services and providers are covered under the member's specific plan

- Checking a claim's status or identifying outstanding expenses

- Working closely with the finance department to process payments and helping direct members who are concerned about their bills to the appropriate and helpful resources

- Acting as the first line of defense against complaints and grievances, and providing information about claim denials and appeals

- Fielding questions from brokers, who are responsible for maintaining the relationship with their employer or government agency clients

As more and more organizations adopt online portals, CSRs also are assisting users with the PSHP's website's self-service functions, including making premium payments, changing an address and resetting passwords.

In conjunction with performing these tasks, CSRs must educate plan members and providers. For some, like experienced providers, this education is minimal. But do not underestimate the operational implications created by your members who need help navigating through their health insurance information.

Case Study:
Learning About Customer Service Demands During the First Year of Affordable Care Act Operations and the Uninitiated Insurance Shopper

"Whether it's a Consumer-Operated-and-Oriented Plan (CO-OP) or an established health plan selling on the exchanges, people buying coverage often were confused by what that meant," says Karen Janousek, President of Health Plan Services, Valence Health. To first-time insurance shoppers, the information coming at them was laced with foreign words and phrases: deductible, co-payment; maximum out of pocket; accumulator formulas. Websites such as HealthCare.gov had explanations that Janousek read and understood, "but I read it as a reader who understands this business." The sheer volume of calls about fundamental aspects of benefit plans took exchange plans by surprise.

Valence Health has other CO-OP clients across the country in addition to Maine Community Health Options (MCHO), who were seeking advice on how to start up their plans and provide the data, analytical and actuarial operational support these organizations need to learn how to work with their providers efficiently and handle financial risk. As Valence Health brought up its health plan's and CO-OP's clients for the open exchange enrollment, "We thought we were overstaffed for customer service, and it turns out, we probably had half the staff we should have had waiting to take those calls," says R. Todd Stockard, President and Co-Founder.

MCHO started with five call center staffers; it's now at 25. Other staff with insurance broker licenses was mobilized for the information crush and executives also manned the enrollment frontlines. "We had a team of anywhere from 20 to 30 on any given day and, even then, that was insufficient at times," says Kevin Lewis, Chief Executive Officer of MCHO.

First, the average two-minute inquiry typical of commercial customer service went five to seven minutes, much of it dealing with the basics of insurance. Then, there were calls a few days later from the same people wanting to have the whole conversation all over again to cement their understanding. Once new members accessed care for the first time, many were on the phone again asking why they got a bill reflecting deductible, co-pay and other cost-sharing — "I thought I was insured."

For the second-year enrollment cycle, much work has gone into developing aids so that health plans can manage inbound call volume better; namely, explanatory language that is easier for the uninitiated to grasp; video clips that promote self-service communications; mailings with simplified diagrams about how the insurance process works; and other step-by-step aids. New rounds bring new issues into the mix; for example, switching plans for the first time and the attendant re-education process, and keeping the members that a plan enrolled the first year. Ongoing success depends on engaging people to become members and renew year after year, and that involves creating an educational dimension that the plans legitimately hope will pay dividends in retention rates for years going forward.

In essence, CSRs will need to provide health insurance 101. What are deductibles? What are copayments? How is that different from coinsurance? Members with commercial plans tend to be more educated on health insurance topics or have had their insurance for a long period of time. They might not need the basics, but likely will need help understanding more complex topics, like prior authorization or an explanation of benefits (EOB). To see frequently asked member-centric EOB questions and CSR responses, see Figure 8.2.

One key to successfully performing these functions is to truly understand the customers' needs and have CSRs who are empathetic and have a positive attitude. Conducting market research through focus groups and interviews with target populations is one way to help you understand what customers want and expect.

This knowledge can be embedded into the CSRs' call scripts and policies, delivered through technology and further reinforced through ongoing training sessions. Regular spot audits also can be used to monitor CSRs' quality and to identify areas needing improvement and areas of excellence. One of the most effective ways to maintain quality service is to track metrics and analyze corresponding data.

At Valence Health, we have found that consistent training, evaluation and monitoring are particularly important because they provide the customer service area, which is generally characterized by high turnover rates and lower pay, with a level of continuity.

Measuring Success through Benchmarking and Performance Metrics

Every call matters. It only takes one poor experience to put a dent in your health plan's reputation and reduce its value in a member's eyes. Therefore, it is important

Explanation of Benefits FAQ

Source: Valence Health

I just received an EOB. Is this a bill?

CSR: No, this is not a bill. The EOB is a notification that is sent to the patient. This notification provides details on a claim submitted by your provider, including the amount that was already paid to the provider and the amount that you still owe the provider.

What amount do I owe the provider?

CSR: The amount you owe the provider is listed under deductible, coinsurance and copayment.

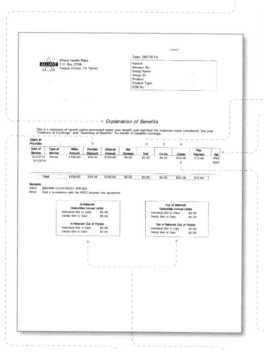

What does the wording under the "Ref" column mean?

CSR: This information is the claim remark code used to identify how the claim was paid. The descriptions of the codes are listed under "Remarks."

Why is there a copay amount on the EOB when I already paid the provider my copay?

CSR: The EOB lists your financial responsibility. If you have already paid your provider the copay shown, then you do not owe any additional copay amount.

Can the provider bill me for the provider discount amount?

CSR: If the provider is within this health plan, then it should not bill you for the provider discount amount. If the provider is outside this plan, then it can bill you for the ineligible amount. You may submit a formal appeal asking this health plan to consider paying the ineligible amount on your behalf, but there is no guarantee of payment.

How much of my deductible has been met?

CSR: The bottom of the EOB lists the current dollar amounts that apply to your deductible. This dollar amount is divided between in-network, out-of-network, individual and family deductibles. Depending on what numbers are here, you may or may not have met all of your deductible obligations.

Figure 8.2

for customer service teams to trend and analyze performance metrics, or key performance indicators (KPIs), so they can assess the department's success and effectiveness. Several commonly tracked metrics are listed as follows:

First Call Resolution (FCR)

The CSR's ability to effectively resolve a caller's questions or concerns on the first attempt is referred to as first call resolution, or FCR. This metric not only monitors how well the callers' issues are resolved, but also indirectly measures the CSR's performance, the customer service area's efficiency and the level of customer satisfaction.

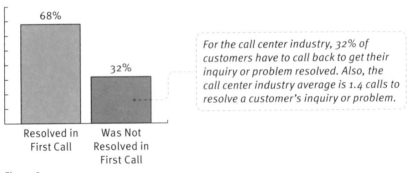

Call Center Industry First Call Resolution Performance

Source: Service Quality Measurement (SQM)

For the call center industry, 32% of customers have to call back to get their inquiry or problem resolved. Also, the call center industry average is 1.4 calls to resolve a customer's inquiry or problem.

Figure 8.3

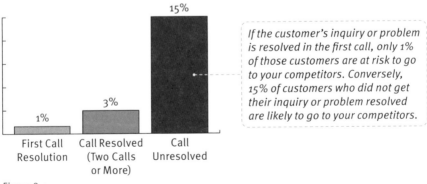

Call Resolution Impact on Customers at Risk

Source: Service Quality Measurement (SQM)

If the customer's inquiry or problem is resolved in the first call, only 1% of those customers are at risk to go to your competitors. Conversely, 15% of customers who did not get their inquiry or problem resolved are likely to go to your competitors.

Figure 8.4

FCR is arguably the most valuable KPI due to its strong correlation with customer satisfaction. If customers do not need to be transferred, call again or wait for a representative to reach out with more information, then they are more likely to perceive the quality of the health plan as high. In general, health plans aim to have at least 80 percent FCR performance and a low percentage of open tickets (unresolved issues). This metric can be captured more accurately by allowing the callers to indicate if their question or concern was resolved through real-time or near-real-time customer survey feedback channels.

Along with an increased customer satisfaction rate, high FCR can facilitate numerous other benefits. With fewer repeat callers, the customer service department can lower its operating costs and improve employee satisfaction. By achieving high FCR, CSRs can feel empowered and confident in their ability to provide quality customer service. Likewise, satisfied customers are more likely to remain loyal, reducing the amount of revenue that is at risk of members defecting to competing health plans.

Service Level (SL)

This speed-of-answer metric identifies the percentage of calls answered in a certain number of seconds. Generally, customer service teams strive to answer 80 percent of the day's calls within 20 or 30 seconds. This type of specific SL objective should also be specified in your PSHP's Service Level Agreement with its ultimate payors. In some Medicaid plans, these SL metrics will be set by the state and your PSHP will have to be able to show its attainment of these metrics.

However, it is critical to not only obtain, but also maintain this goal. CSRs need to consistently monitor and reach SL expectations, even when challenges occur such as understaffing, unusually high call volumes or unexpected service outages. For your plan, these KPIs also will help you to develop customer service budgets and determine resource allocation. These KPIs will be helpful when your plan adds or retires products to understand some operational downstream impacts.

Average Wait Time

This metric tracks the average amount of time that passes before CSRs answer incoming calls. Rather than evaluating an individual CSR's performance, this KPI is typically used to evaluate the entire team's performance and efficiency. If callers wait for what they perceive to be an unacceptable amount of time, then they are more likely to become frustrated and shift their loyalty to a competitor, negatively impacting your organization's revenue.

Abandonment Rate

The percentage of callers who hang up or are disconnected prior to connecting with a CSR is called the abandonment rate. In general, the higher the average wait time, the higher the abandonment rate. Therefore, most organizations use both these metrics to assess customer service performance, and subsequently create an environment that reduces both abandonment and wait times, while improving the customer experience.

Call Handling Time

This KPI measures the amount of time required to resolve the customer's questions or concerns, including any corresponding administrative duties that are need to resolve the issue or move it on to the next stage of resolution. This provides information about the efficiency of both individual CSRs and the customer service area as a whole. However, this metric will fluctuate depending upon each call's nature and complexity, so the more calls that are averaged, the more accurate the metric.

Idle Time

This metric tracks how much time CSRs take to complete required business and administrative tasks related to a call. These necessary tasks may include submitting call reports or compiling and mailing a caller's requested material. The amount of time required will vary depending upon the call, but it can provide insights about each CSR's individual efficiency. Customer service areas strive to maintain reasonably low idle time because this allows CSRs to spend more time directly engaged with customers.

Adherence to Schedule

This time-management KPI measures the amount of time CSRs are performing or available for work activities, including interacting with customers, completing administrative tasks and waiting for incoming calls. This KPI also takes into account numerous other metrics such as number of calls answered, call handling time and average wait time. As many of these previous metrics are outside of the CSR's control, adherence to schedule has become an increasingly valuable KPI for its ability to identify if a staff member is in the right place at the right time.

Organizations generally desire adherence rates between 80 percent and 90 percent because this suggests that CSRs are performing cost-effective, high-quality work. Failure to reach this goal also may indicate an inability to meet the terms in the customer's Service Level Agreement. Organizations that choose to track this metric must be mindful of their staff's needs and abilities.

Adherence to schedule is not intended to encourage micromanagement, and it is important that staff have adequate time for breaks, lunch and training. For this reason, it is typically unrealistic for organizations to set adherence rates between 90 percent and 100 percent.

Expert Insight

"We are very fortunate that so many provider organizations have entrusted some or all of their customer service support needs to Valence Health. As a result, we are able to share best practices and lessons learned quickly and efficiently.

Whenever we pick up the phone or answer an email on behalf of one of our clients, we strike a professional and compassionate balance between the member's needs, the health plan's guidelines and the provider's desires. We also are able to maintain a level of objectivity in helping with the CSR role so that if we see operational trends or issues expressing themselves via the calls and emails we are handling, our staff can elevate those issues and help our client's leadership team take informed and decisive action.

Through these partnerships, we really know that our job is to help advance the mission of our PSHP by being an extension of their customer service team."

– Phil Kamp
CEO and Co-Founder, Valence Health

The industry at large has no lack of metrics for tracking customer service performance. In addition to the seven common KPIs mentioned above, there are numerous other metrics for factors like hold time, transfer rate, ratio of active to waiting calls, overall number of inbound calls, total answered calls and staff turnover rate. All of these metrics impact the quality of the CSR-customer interactions and overall customer satisfaction. ⊘

Tracking Key Health Plan Customer Service Metrics

Performing regular data analysis can help your PSHP maximize its return on investment and identify both early warning signs of trouble and indicators of success. By tracking key inputs and outputs, you can continually enhance your health plan so it retains members, remains financially stable and earns high patient satisfaction scores. Below are key customer service metrics that should be measured continuously:

- Customer retention rate
- Frequency of CSR-customer communication via phone, email and online chat
- Frequency and type of CSR communication with providers, members and brokers
- Adoption rate of online portals
- Number of grievances and complaints
- Market research results from focus groups, customer surveys, etc.
- CSR spot audits results
- First call resolution (FCR) rate
- Number of repeat callers
- Number of open tickets
- Operating costs
- CSR employee satisfaction surveys
- Service level (SL) percentage
- Daily "valleys and peaks" in call and online chat volumes
- Resource allocation
- Customer service level of accessibility
- Average wait time
- Individual CSR performance
- Overall customer service area performance
- Abandonment rate
- Call handling time
- Idle time
- Adherence to schedule
- Total answered calls
- Hold time
- Transfer rate
- Ratio of active to waiting calls
- Total inbound calls per CSR and as a group
- Total outbound calls per and as a group
- Customer satisfaction surveys

Industry Terminology Related to Customer Service

Benefit   A service covered by a member's health insurance.

Source: The California Department of Managed Healthcare

Claim   A request for payment that you or your healthcare provider submits to your health insurer when you get items or services you think are covered.

Source: Healthcare.gov

Eligibility   Entitlement of an individual to receive services based on that individual's enrollment in a healthcare plan.

Source: Mosby's Medical Dictionary, 8th edition

Explanation of Benefits (EOB)   A statement sent by a health insurance company to covered individuals explaining what medical treatments and/or services were paid for on their behalf.

Source: Valence Health

Grievance   A grievance is any complaint or dispute (other than an organization determination) expressing dissatisfaction with any aspect of the operations, activities or behavior of a health plan or its providers, regardless of whether remedial action is requested. The enrollee must file the grievance either orally or in writing no later than 60 days after the triggering event or incident precipitating the grievance.

Source: CMS.gov

Open Enrollment   A period of time, usually but not always occurring once per year, when employees of companies and organizations may make changes to their elected fringe benefit options, such as health insurance. The term also applies to the annual period during which individuals may buy individual health insurance plans through the online, state-based health insurance exchanges established by the Patient Protection and Affordable Care Act.

Source: Wikipedia.org

Premium   The amount that must be paid by the insured for his/her health insurance or plan. The member or his/her employers usually pay the premium monthly, quarterly or yearly.

Source: HealthCare.gov

Prior Authorization   Approval from a health plan that may be required before a member gets a service or fills a prescription in order for the service or prescription to be covered by their plan.

Source: HealthCare.gov

Chapter Nine
Claims Administration and Management

A critical, but not very glamorous role of any insurance company is to process and adjudicate claims. So as you get ready to fully operationalize your provider-sponsored health plan (PSHP), you will need to know how your plan will both create and maintain processes that pay claims as smoothly and accurately as possible. If your plan can do this faster and more accurately and seamlessly than your competitors, you also have the chance to create greater reasons for other local healthcare providers to join your network. This also can be a key differentiator when trying to sell your plans to individuals, employers, brokers and government agencies.

The less time and energy your ultimate payors have to devote to resolving healthcare claim issues or taking complaints from their employees and beneficiaries about these critical payment issues (in the case of commercial, Medicare and Medicaid plans), the more time they will have to do other more value-added activities. In short, if you relieve potential claims headaches for your payors, they will come to truly appreciate that you have a better health plan.

> **Expert Insight**
>
> *"What I have seen is that processing claims comes down to the real basic fundamentals. Usually the health plans that struggle are the ones that are missing some of the core fundamentals."*
>
> **– Anthony Gutierrez**
> Vice President of Operations, Valence Health

Claims administration and management are very technical parts of the health plan business. They also represent very significant investments in technology as it is essential to automate the largest portions of these processes in ways that reduce mistakes and create crystal clear records for payors, members and healthcare providers (for more information about critical claims processing technology refer to Chapter 12, "Health Plan Technology").

> **Expert Insight**
>
> *"When we began helping providers pay claims — both PSHPs and other folks who had accepted that responsibility as part of a capitated contracting situation — we had to make our own build, buy or partner/outsource decision about our core technology.*
>
> *After evaluating the claims-processing platforms available on the market, we entered into a strategic partnership with Aldera to take its core system and adapt it to the unique needs of our provider clients. This has allowed both of our organizations to scale over time in ways that uniquely address the needs of our own Valence Health staff, the staff of many of our clients, the members of their health plans and the providers who deliver care."*
>
> **– R. Todd Stockard**
> President and Co-Founder, Valence Health

In the end, each of these key stakeholders is intimately impacted by your PSHP's decision to accept or reject each claim. A paid claim means funds flow into a provider's office or institution. A rejected claim may mean that individual members will have to pay for something themselves out of their own pocket or risk ruining their credit rating if they fail to do so. Therefore, the decision to build, buy or partner/outsource when it comes to claims administration and management probably will be one of the biggest executional strategy decisions your leadership team will make (refer to Chapter 3 for more about "Determining Your PSHP's Comprehensive Execution Strategy").

You also need to be very aware that all of your other health plan competitors will have wrestled with and come up with solutions to address their claims administration and management needs. They know that as a start-up, with less traditional insurance experience, this will be a huge new operational roadblock for your PSHP to resolve.

Therefore, to help truly inform your build, buy or partner/outsource decision specifically around claims administration and management, we have devoted the rest of this chapter to the technical and detailed aspects of what goes into establishing and maintaining the business rules that will become the backbone of these critical processes.

To do this, you need to start with the basic fundamentals because if any member of your organization makes a mistake in adjudicating the claim, then the system cannot process it. To start, there are a few things you need to understand, including reimbursement models and code sets.

Reimbursement Models and Code Sets

You need to know the rules of the road before you can drive safely and running your PSHP is no different. You need to know the rules surrounding reimbursement models and code sets before you can write contracts, process claims and calculate reimbursements properly. The rules you must abide by will vary depending upon what type of plans you offer.

Generally speaking, Medicare and other plans that are associated with the government have a strict, clear set of rules outlined in their contracts. For example, Medicare has pre-determined fee schedules that specify how much each provider will get paid for performing specific medical services. Neither the provider nor your organization has any real input on this topic. You simply need to understand the government's rules and design your internal claims system in a way that can correctly process the claims and meet associated deadlines (for more information on claims technology, refer to Chapter 12, "Health Plan Technology").

For other commercial plan offerings, however, you will determine the reimbursement models and any corresponding fee schedules yourself. While your PSHP can choose to base its commercial reimbursement models off of government models, the choice will be yours. As outlined in Chapter 6, "Network Development and Management," value-based reimbursement models (see Figure 9.1) offer your PSHP the chance to align financial opportunities and incentives in ways that you think will have the greatest positive impact on your plan's membership. In the end, it is up to your organization to negotiate a contract with a fair reimbursement model and fee schedule as appropriate (for more information on developing network contracts, refer to the same chapter).

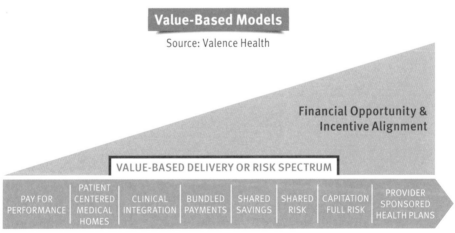

Value-Based Models

Source: Valence Health

Financial Opportunity & Incentive Alignment

VALUE-BASED DELIVERY OR RISK SPECTRUM

| PAY FOR PERFORMANCE | PATIENT CENTERED MEDICAL HOMES | CLINICAL INTEGRATION | BUNDLED PAYMENTS | SHARED SAVINGS | SHARED RISK | CAPITATION FULL RISK | PROVIDER SPONSORED HEALTH PLANS |

Figure 9.1

So if you are wondering how rendered services and procedures get uniformly described and subsequently translated into accurate reimbursement, the answer is code sets.

Under the Health Insurance Portability and Accountability Act of 1996 (HIPAA), the Department of Health and Human Services (HHS) adopted specific code sets to be used when listing rendered services that will be submitted for reimbursement. This practice helps ensure claims are adjudicated in a consistent manner. The standardized code sets include Current Procedural Terminology (CPT), the International Classification of Diseases (ICD) and Healthcare Common Procedure Coding System (HCPCS).

With approximately 7,800 codes, the CPT codes are used to clearly describe the medical, surgical and diagnostic services or procedures conducted by physicians and other healthcare providers. These numeric codes are five digits long and may contain a two-digit modifier if additional clarity is needed. The American Medical Association developed and copyrighted the CPT codes and continues to update them annually.

In addition to CPT codes, three-digit ICD codes are used to uniformly identify a diagnosis, disease, disorder or medical condition. These two code sets must support one another, meaning the procedure must align with the diagnosis. This code set is maintained in the U.S. by the National Center for Health Statistics of the Centers for Disease Control and Prevention.

HCPCS also are connected closely with CPT codes. Used by Medicare, this code set has two levels: Level I consists of all CPT codes, while Level II is an alphanumeric code set that describes a variety of products, supplies and services that are not included in the CPT codes. This allows claims to be billed for services like ambulance services and durable medical equipment, prosthetics, orthotics and supplies when used outside a physician's office, which cannot be described using CPT codes alone. The Level II code set is maintained by the Centers for Medicare & Medicaid Services (CMS) and is revised quarterly using feedback from multiple sources, including providers, manufacturers, vendors, payors, government agencies and specialty societies.

In addition to these standard code sets, specific revenue codes are required by payors to identify where procedures were performed. As outlined in a health plan's contract with other healthcare providers, these four-digit codes can affect reimbursement because the identical service may receive different reimbursement rates depending on if it was provided in the emergency room, operating room or maternity ward, for example. Revenue codes also group similar types of charges onto one line in the claim.

Code sets are necessary when calculating provider payment because they form the fundamental equations that make consistent, accurate reimbursement possible.

The Medicare Physician Fee Schedule (PFS) is used to determine uniform physician payment rates for specific services and procedures on a fee-for-service basis. The list of rendered services are coded using HCPCS, with each CPT code assigned a corresponding Relative Value Unit (RVU). These RVUs are used to take into account three cost factors associated with providing medical services:

- The physician work RVU represents the relative amount of time, skill, training and intensity required by a service. The higher the RVU, the more demanding the service

- The practice expense (PE) RVU reflects the financial costs of running a practice, such as the direct and indirect expenses associated with rent, equipment, supplies and staff

- The malpractice (MP) RVU addresses professional liability costs

The RVU Scale Update Committee contains experts who periodically review the RVUs and make adjustment recommendations to CMS.

To calculate appropriate reimbursement, each of the three RVUs is adjusted for geographic differences in cost using the Geographic Practice Cost Indices (GPCI). The GPCI is updated every three years. Separate GPCIs also are developed for each Medicare payment location and for each of the three RVUs. The formula for calculating Medicare PFS payment rates (see Figure 9.2) requires each RVU to be multiplied by its corresponding GPCI and then added together. The total is then multiplied by the national Conversion Factor (CF), which converts the complex total into a tangible dollar amount. This amount, pending any additional adjustments for extraneous factors, is covered primarily by Medicare with a smaller portion becoming the member's out-of-pocket expense.

Medicare Physician Fee Schedule Payment Rates Formula

Source: HHS, CMS and Medicare Learning Network

$$\text{Payment} = \left[\text{Work RVU} \times \text{Work GPCI} + \text{PE RVU} \times \text{PE GPCI} + \text{MP RVU} \times \text{MP GPCI} \right] \times \text{CF}$$

Figure 9.2

In addition to reimbursing providers using the Medicare PFS, Medicare reimburses hospitals for inpatient services using the Inpatient Prospective Payment System (IPPS) and for outpatient services using the Hospital Outpatient Prospective Payment System (OPPS).

IPPS rates are designed to control hospital costs by issuing pre-determined reimbursement amounts for the expected expenses that efficient hospitals will incur for specific services. This means that rather than paying hospitals for every day of service or each piece of medical equipment used, Medicare pays based on the patient's diagnosis. To do this, Medicare specifies standardized payment rates that account for the efficient operating and capital costs incurred when hospitals provide medical care. These base rates are then adjusted to reflect costs associated with the local market or geographic factors and the patient's condition.

Medicare used the wage index, a tool used to measure differences in local salary rates, to account for market and geographic factors, as well as the medical severity diagnosis related group (MS-DRG) system (which is based on ICD codes) to group patients with similar medical conditions. Each MS-DRG has an assigned weight that correlates with the average cost of treatment and resource utilization for patients in that group. These MS-DRG weights are updated annually by CMS to account for new diagnoses or information, and to ensure the MS-DRGs only contain conditions with similar costs.

Due to the success of MS-DRGs, CMS implemented OPPS in August 2000. To calculate payment in OPPS, services are coded using HCPCS. Next, HCPCS with similar clinical aspects and resource utilization are grouped into different ambulatory payment classifications (APCs). Each APC has a fixed reimbursement amount that is intended to control medical costs while providing sufficient reimbursement. APC payments are issued when Medicare outpatient members are transferred to an unaffiliated hospital or discharged from a clinic or emergency department. CMS consults with a panel of outside experts annually to update the APCs by reviewing new services or cost data, changes in technology or medical practices and other relevant information.

Although Medicare physician fee, outpatient fee and inpatient fee schedules are associated with government reimbursement, commercial payors frequently use similar components. For this reason, it is common for commercial contracts to reflect RVUs, APCs or other key concepts in their reimbursement structure.

In addition, out-of-network providers who deliver care are primarily reimbursed under the Maximum Non-Network Reimbursement Program (MNRP), which bases payments on a percentage of the schedule rates allowed by Medicare. Since out-of-network providers do not have contractual agreements that provide health plans discounted fees to reduce the cost of medical services, this program limits the maximum expenses (see Figure 9.3).

Maximum Non-Network Reimbursement Program Examples*

Source: UnitedHealthcare

Physician Office Visit Claim		
	Network	Non-Network
A: Billed Charge Amount	$270	$270
B: Eligible Expense (amount UnitedHealthcare allows)	Paid per Contract	$1,740 (MNRP Pricing)
C: Network Copay/30% Non-Network Coinsurance	$20	$45 (30% of B)
D: Additional Enrollee Responsibility	$0	$120**
Enrollee Financial Responsibility	$20	$165

Facility Claim		
	Network	Non-Network
A: Billed Charge Amount	$3,700	$3,700
B: Eligible Expense (amount UnitedHealthcare allows)	Paid per Contract	$1,740 (MNRP Pricing)
C: Network Copay/30% Non-Network Coinsurance	$500	$522 (30% of B)
D: Additional Enrollee Responsibility	$0	$1,960**
Enrollee Financial Responsibility	$500	$2,482

MNRP=Maximum Non-Network Reimbursement Program
*Please note these examples are for illustration only.
**This amount does not apply to the out-of-pocket maximum.
Figure 9.3

Contract Rules

Your PSHP's reimbursement models and code sets need to be fully outlined in the contracts you put in place with your network providers. These contracts also will have to cover rules on a wide variety of topics including the conditions, limitations and exclusions of the agreement. It is critical to write comprehensive, clear contracts because these documents ultimately determine what does and does not get paid.

- **Conditions**
  The conditions explain the requirements and procedures that certain parties must follow. For example, contracts contain patient eligibility and enrollment information, including expectations surrounding premium payments. They also clarify steps in the billing process and the acceptable timeline for specific billing and collection events. Your plan will need to state if electronic and/or paper billing is acceptable and set

timely filing requirements, which dictate the number of days allowed for claim submission. The timeframe your health plan has for processing the claims and making payments also must be specified along with the process and timeframe allowed when submitting appeals for denied claims. Contracts also generally contain numerous other conditions, including nondiscrimination clauses, prior authorization information and notification requirements for any policy changes.

- **Limitations**

  Contract limitations outline the policy's boundaries, including members' coverage restrictions regarding how often healthcare services and treatments can be performed and over what time period. For example, your plan may only allow providers to bill for an annual physical once every 12 months, but no sooner than the service date of last year's physical. The limitations also address the plan's maximum payment amounts and the members' cost-sharing arrangements (for more information on cost-sharing arrangements, refer to Chapter 4, "Plan Design"). Other important items include the contract's term, renegotiation and termination agreements about the length of the contract and how to reopen or close it.

- **Exclusions**

  Contracts also include exclusions about what is outside the agreement's scope. For example, your PSHP may not cover certain services, such as experimental or cosmetic treatments. Likewise, not all healthcare professionals are in-network and provide discounted fees.

If a claim does not meet the rules for payment that are laid out in the contracts you have set up with your network providers, as the payor, your PSHP can deny all or part of the claim. This prevents your PSHP from paying claims that are outside your scope, but it may require a member or healthcare organization to cover more of the claim expense. Therefore, it is critical that all parties involved understand the contract's conditions, limitations and exclusions.

Unfortunately, sometimes contracts are ambiguous or staff members simply make mistakes and do not process claims correctly. For this reason, you will need an audit and recovery function. The purpose of this function is to catch and correct errors post-payment to collect what would otherwise be lost revenue. Individuals who work in this area often perform post-audit reviews of accounts to verify that the procedures and rules outlined in your PSHP's contracts with various network providers were followed correctly and that accurate reimbursements were issued.

For example, audit and recovery professionals often look at claims like auto accidents to determine if a different entity should actually be paying the bill or if your plan paid too much. Alternatively, audit and recovery professionals may realize that certain healthcare services were not actually performed. If a mistake is found, the recovery department can collect this money and process refund checks.

Premium Billing

Another task your PSHP will need to manage is premium billing. This is the process of delivering bills to employers, individual members or to government agencies — depending upon your type of plan — so that premium payments can be collected. Since all health plans' primary source of income comes from premium billing, this will be a critical function for making sure there is enough gas to run your PSHP.

To drive premium billing, your PSHP needs to accurately identify all eligible members for each of its different plans or products. This of course will differ somewhat given the types of products your PSHP have chosen to offer or sell.

If your PSHP has plans that you offer directly to individuals, both on and off public and private exchanges, your claims administration and management system will create an account that includes a description of the individuals' benefit package levels and dependent information. As part of this account, your system also will note the corresponding premium amounts that were established when the individual member enrolled in your plan. The billing statements, or invoices, list the total account balance for the applicable eligibility period and the minimum payment due.

For individual purchasers, the bills are delivered directly to the enrollee with details about the individual and their dependents so that the enrollee can individually make a payment. Depending upon your plan's policies, these payments can be accepted via online bill pay, automatic bank withdrawals, mailed payments or in-person transactions. The timing for this billing also is at your discretion, meaning you can bill individual members once a month, four times a year, etc.

If your PSHP is providing health insurance to a group of individuals via employers, Medicare or Medicaid, the payor (i.e., the employer, CMS and/or the state Medicaid agency) will receive and pay these bills. Group bills will contain information on all of the employees or beneficiaries (in the case of Medicare and Medicaid) and any of their dependents that are covered under these accounts or groups.

To ensure your plan's enrollment records are accurate and payments can be collected effectively, both individuals and groups must promptly communicate to your plan any and all changes in a member's health insurance status. For example, these kinds of changes will include things like adjustments in individual coverage options, or terminated or newly enrolled members and dependents. Without this critically important eligibility information, your plan runs the risk of both overpaying and denying claims for members who may or may not be covered by one of your PSHP's products.

The highly dynamic nature of this data makes changing eligibility a common headache in the healthcare insurance industry, and for Valence Health's PSHP clients that decided to offer products on the state and federal exchanges. These plans experience frequent membership status changes, especially between exchange and Medicaid coverage.

For example, in month one, a person may be covered by exchange insurance, but after a job loss or the birth of a child, he or she is then Medicaid-eligible in months two through four. If the member goes back to work in month five, he or she loses Medicaid coverage and is again eligible for exchange coverage. Alternatively, a parent may retain public exchange coverage, but his/her children are eligible for Medicaid. For our clients that have both an exchange and a Medicaid product, they have been able to deliver uniquely coordinated and uninterrupted level of healthcare service and coverage for the families and providers who are impacted by these real economic situations.

Another common and complex eligibility situation occurs when your plan's members switch to or add a new insurance company. When members change their insurance coverage, your plan will need to refer to its contract with the payor to determine how to finance the patient's continuity of care. For example, if the member's coverage changes while the patient is hospitalized, pregnant or receiving behavioral health services, your plan must identify if or when it will stop paying for these medical expenses.

Likewise, some of you plan's members will add another insurance plan for themselves or a dependent. In these scenarios, your plan will need to determine which insurance company pays for claims first by establishing and following rules for the proper coordination of benefits (COB). In the commercial market, some of your members may have their own insurance and secondary insurance through a spouse or partner. In these situations, you need to know when your plan will be the first payor or the secondary payor. In Medicaid for example, CMS has a set of rules that establish Medicaid as the payor of last resort and it helps health plans determine when Medicare will be the secondary payor. Therefore, your PSHP's contracts will need to contain its own COB program with a set of rules for determining primary and secondary coverage.

Another unfortunate but common issue in premium billing is lack of payment. Unfortunately, some members fail to make timely payments, are unable to afford payments or disregard their financial obligations. In the case of government contracts, these payments may be delayed. For example, a state budget that has not yet been finalized impacts the timeliness in which your Medicaid premium may arrive. Contracts generally allow members a finite period of time, called a grace period, to make late premium payments before their coverage is terminated. During this timeframe, health plans often set up payments plans, send past due notices and perform other follow-up activities in an attempt to collect payment.

At the same time, providers and healthcare organizations should be notified, according to specifications in the contract, when the member enters the premium payment grace period. This practice allows healthcare organizations to inquire with patients or your health plan about coverage status prior to delivering non-emergent medical services. Any services that are rendered during this grace period will need to be paid according to the terms of the contract. ⊘

Tracking Key Health Plan Claims Administration and Management Metrics

Performing regular data analysis can help your PSHP maximize its return on investment and identify both early warning signs of trouble and indicators of success. By tracking key inputs and outputs, you can continually enhance your health plan so it retains members, remains financially stable and earns high patient satisfaction scores. Below are key claims administration and management metrics that should be measured continuously:

- Number of errors in adjudicating claims
- Lists of providers who consistently or more regularly have coding errors
- Your plan's commercial payment rates
- Medicare payment rates
- Medicaid payment rates
- Maximum Non-Network Reimbursement Program payment rates
- Practice expenses incurred by network providers
- Network's malpractice costs
- Geographic differences in cost
- Average cost of treatment and resource utilization for specific services

- New medical cost information
- Number of denied claims
- Number and status of appealed claims and denials
- Audit and recovery collections amount
- Amount of lost premium dollars
- Number of members
- Frequency of changing eligibility
- Number of payments made during the grace period
- Provider notification policy for late premium payments
- Number of claims with services rendered during grace periods

Industry Terminology Related to Claims Administration and Management

Appeal   A request for your health insurer or plan to review a decision or a grievance again.

Source: HealthCare.gov

Claim Adjudication   The determination of the insurer's payment or financial responsibility after the member's insurance benefits are applied to a medical claim.

Source: Medicaloffice.about.com

Continuity of Care   Continuity of care is concerned with quality of care over time. It is the process by which the patient and his/her physician-led care team are cooperatively involved in ongoing healthcare management toward the shared goal of high quality, cost-effective medical care.

Source: American Academy of Family Physicians

Coordination of Benefits (COB)   A way to figure out who pays first when two or more health insurance plans are responsible for paying the same medical claim.

Source: HealthCare.gov

Cost-Sharing   The share of costs covered by the member's insurance that the member pays out of his/her own pocket. This term generally includes deductibles, coinsurance and copayments or similar charges, but it does not include premiums, balance billing amounts for non-network providers or the cost of non-covered services. Cost-sharing in Medicaid and the Children's Health Insurance Program also includes premiums.

Source: HealthCare.gov

Denied Claim   The refusal of an insurance company or carrier to honor a request by an individual (or his or her provider) to pay for healthcare services obtained from a healthcare professional.

Source: Healthinsurance.org

Premium   The amount that must be paid by the insured for his/her health insurance or plan. The member or his/her employers usually pay the premium monthly, quarterly or yearly.

Source: HealthCare.gov

Primary Coverage   If a person is covered under more than one health insurance plan, primary coverage is the coverage provided by the health insurance plan that pays on claims first.

Source: eHealth

Prior Authorization   Approval from a health plan that may be required before members get a service or fills a prescription in order for the service or prescription to be covered by their plan.

Source: HealthCare.gov

Secondary Coverage   When a person is covered under more than one health insurance plan, this term describes the health insurance plan that provides payment on claims after the primary coverage.

Source: eHealth

Chapter Ten
Actuarial Considerations and Financial Management

The undeniable truth about any business is that it cannot succeed without sufficient financing or a viable cost structure. Otherwise, no matter how perfect your health plan is, your provider-sponsored health plan (PSHP) will run out of gas and be unable to go anywhere.

The ability to start a PSHP is largely driven by two factors: cash on-hand and the state of your balance sheet. To determine the liquidity of your PSHP's affiliated healthcare organization, you can pull items like your financial statements, balance sheets and credit reports. But before you can know for certain if you are in the financial position to create a PSHP, you need to have an honest talk with an actuarial team to learn how much capital you need.

Actuarial Considerations

At the end of the day, insurance is a risk. To assess risk in the insurance field and other industries, the discipline of actuarial science uses mathematical and statistical methods to identify, evaluate and advise on how to best prepare for uncertain future events. This includes a variety of applications from analyzing mortality and creating life tables in the life insurance industry, to assessing employee benefit plans and monitoring social welfare programs for various government agencies.

The job of actuarial services in the health insurance field is to help organizations, like yours, mitigate their risk and protect their soundness. So what is your organization's insurance risk and how should you manage it? The only way to find out is with data and supporting analytics.

To calculate insurance risk, actuaries will need demographic and geographic information, along with illness burden and consumer behavior for your potential members. Hopefully, you will have much of this information through a combination of data sources like your provider members, electronic medical records, practice management systems or your community health information exchange. To update this

> ### Expert Insight
>
> *"The most important asset for any actuary is data. People want to talk about really cool logistical trending and regression analysis — and we do some of that — but the starting point for everything an actuary does revolves around accessing relevant information and data."*
>
> **– Steve Tutewohl**
> Strategic Accounts Officer, Valence Health

information for patients who are already seeing providers in one of your PSHP's parent organizations or to gather this information from new enrollees, many plans use a health risk assessment (HRA). Some plans also have customer service representatives ask their members questions about HRAs when they call or interact online for another reason.

The HRA is an objective tool that can be used to calculate each enrollee's risk score. This self-assessment contains a variety of questions about the factors that impact insurance risk, including the patient's demographics, current and past medical conditions, family history, treatment information and previous healthcare spending. Using algorithms, health plans calculate each individual's numeric risk score and consequently the risk of the entire member population.

Calculating your plan's insurance risk is critical because it can quantify your plan's deviation from the average population's risk. This can potentially translate into additional reimbursement by increasing the capitation rate for members who have a higher stratified level of risk and, therefore, are more likely to have higher-than-average healthcare expenses. As part of the Affordable Care Act (ACA), new rules were enacted that impact all commercial, Medicare and Medicaid health insurance products. Therefore, it is vital that your PSHP team has a deep understanding of the government's various reimbursement programs because it can significantly impact your organization's balance sheet and ultimate profitability (see the Risk Mitigation Strategies sidebar for more details).

Risk Mitigation Strategies:
The 3 R's

With the media regularly reporting new progress toward the adoption of value-based care, how will your PSHP manage in a system that is heavily dominated by value-based payments? To succeed, it is critical for your organization to understand what government reimbursement programs are available for your type of products and how those will impact your pricing and balance sheet.

The options available to you will continually change as new legislation is approved and past legislation ends. With the passage of the ACA, multiple new risk and market stability programs were introduced to supplement past programs and, inevitably, more legislation will be enacted in the decades to come.

Below are three common programs that are available in 2015:

- The risk adjustment program is designed to distribute financial risk across the various plan offerings in the individual and small group insurance markets. The goal is to stabilize plan premiums by discouraging insurers from designing plans that are more appealing to healthier populations. To do this, enrollees' individual risk scores are evaluated to calculate each participating plan's average actuarial risk. Plans that have low-risk members must then make payments to plans with higher-risk members. This permanent program began in 2014.

- The temporary reinsurance program is available for certain plans from 2014 to 2016. Like the risk adjustment program, this initiative aims to stabilize premiums; however, it does this by minimizing the insurer's desire to increase premiums in the wake of the ACA position against preexisting condition exclusions. Under this program, individual market plans that must abide by the new market rules are eligible for payments. The government supports this program by collecting funds from all insurers and third-party administrators, and then distributing them to qualifying plans. Payment amounts are distributed based on where the enrollees' cost falls within a predetermined range.

- The risk corridor program is another temporary option that stems from the ACA. Designed to prevent Qualified Health Plans (QHPs) from incurring large gains or losses, this program incentivizes plans on the Exchange to set appropriate premiums. The government sets a target amount of costs for each QHP's actual claims, which is based on the plan's premium. If a QHP's actual claims are more than plus or minus 3 percent from this target amount, then the QHP will receive payments or be charged, respectively. This program, which extends from 2014 through 2016, encourages QHPs to stay within this allowable range.

Data from the last year is the best way to predict what will happen this upcoming year. And the more data your actuaries have, the more accurate and refined their predictions can be. If you know how last year's services — or the last five years of services — led to claims and payments, then your actuaries can use trending to project that into the future. Unfortunately for new PSHPs, that data will be absent.

With the help of predictive models and analytical tools, your actuaries can use data from various sources to predict the future and tell you the best way — statistically — to prepare for it (for common risk mitigation tactics, see Figure 10.1). Maybe your plans should be priced a certain way or perhaps offer specific medical cost management programs to high-risk members (for more information on medical cost management, refer to Chapter 7, "Medical Management").

Common Risk Mitigation Tactics by Health Insurance Companies

Source: Society of Actuaries

- Identifying diversification or selective participation in exchanges by state or product or customer segment for carriers with broader product lines and in diverse geographic areas
- Communicating with regulators and legislators
- Improving rate filings and pricing changes
- Modifying plan design
- Changing provider contracting and network
- Increasing medical management
- Performing expense management

Figure 10.1

Reserves

Actuaries play a vital role in financial management functions, including calculating how much money your organization needs to place in reserve. These reserves are liquid assets that are earmarked against specific liabilities or money your plan will need to pay out immediately or in the future.

Insurance contracts are essentially a promise to pay, but this promise is only useful if there is money to support it (e.g., gas in your PSHP "bus" tank). For this reason, your PSHP must pledge part of its capital in the form of liquid assets to the state where you operate. This is called a statutory reserve. While this usually is not a large sum of money, it is enough to provide some protection against potential losses. It also is the minimum capital, or reserve of liquid assets, required by the state to begin operating as a health plan.

This type of reserve is essentially a deposit that cannot be used by your organization without permission; however, it will still be part of your overall capital and appear as an asset on your balance sheet. The amount of reserves vary by state and sometimes from product to product within a state, so your best bet is to have your actuary calculate this reserve amount given your plan offering and according to your state's specific requirements.

Along with this statutory reserve, your health plan also is required to have incurred but not reported (IBNR) reserves. These reserves are a liability because they are for services that already have been delivered or rendered, but have not been reported yet. Essentially, the IBNR reserve acknowledges that your plan has a cash need, which must be adjusted every month to match your future expenses.

Relating it to your lovely new PSHP bus, you know there will be expenses, whether they be gas, registration or repairs, so you will set aside money to fund the services you need to cover. If some of these services have already occurred and are simply placed on your credit card, you need to have the reserves in your bank account to cover these services when the bill comes due.

For a health plan, these future expenses take the form of claims. Oftentimes, these claims are still in a queue to be processed, which means your plan must guess what its future expenses will be. As this expense increases, your organization's capital decreases due to the negative equity.

The amount of money placed in these reserves is calculated by actuaries using three main indicators: number of lives, amount of premiums and level of risk. This means that if you are insuring 25,000 Medicaid lives, then you might need $2 million in reserves, while a plan with 100,000 Medicare Advantage lives might need $20 million. This reserve amount also may vary based on how aggressively or conservatively your plans are priced.

Risk-Based Capital

To legally run a health plan, there is one specific hurdle your organization needs to clear: risk-based capital (RBC). This capital requirement is used by the government to make sure that all insurance companies have the minimum amount of capital necessary to offset their amount of risk. This risk includes asset risk, underwriting risk, credit risk and the business risk of your organization. Effectively, this requirement acts as a cushion against insolvency by requiring higher-risk health plans to have more capital and protects patients and providers from health insurance companies going out of business with no way to pay their bills. RBC requirements are standardized by the National Association of Insurance Commissioners (NAIC), but implemented by the state where you operate. For this reason, the requirements vary.

To calculate your RBC, the NAIC provides formulas that are used to project your organization's risk, expenses, expected revenue and payment ability. This will set your organization's minimum net equity level. This formula will be used to fill out the RBC report that will be submitted to your state insurance regulator to justify your risk-based capital levels. This annual report is most difficult to complete in the first year because you will not have historical data, but it will become easier and more accurate in subsequent years.

If the content of your RBC report shows your organization has fallen below the minimum capital requirement, then you are alerted to the problem and given the chance to fix it. There are four levels of action — company action, regulatory action, authorized control and mandatory control levels — that might be required by the regulator, your organization, or both.

For example, if your organization's report triggers the company action level, then you must find a way to restore your capital to normal RBC levels. This could be done by reducing the health plan's membership, pursuing risk mitigation strategies or attaining more capital through a PSHP owner or a third party. The advantage of this setup is that it allows for quick corrective or preventative action that saves your organization from insolvency with minimal court involvement.

Financial Management

To ensure your PSHP does not run out of gas, several key financial management functions must be performed. One of these is accounting. All the financial transactions that occur in your health plan will be tracked and recorded by members of your accounting team. This includes all accounts receivable and accounts payable — or money that is owed to you or by you, respectively. The other set of financial management functions you will need relate to maintaining your plan's general ledger (see Figure 10.2). Again the decision to build, buy or partner/outsource some or all of your financial management functions should be addressed as part of your "Comprehensive Execution Strategy," as outlined in Chapter 3.

Essential Health Plan Accounting and General Ledger Needs

Source: Valence Health

- Send invoices
- Collect accounts receivable
- Review payments owed
- Issue expense reports and statements
- Conduct audits
- Reconcile and submit bank statements
- Reconcile and submit federal report-ins
- File state and federal taxes
- Administer payroll system with support from human resources
- Establish and maintain banking relationships for both collection and payment activities
- Liaison between your plan and any agencies performing financial audits (for more information on compliance, financial auditing and statutory and federal reporting, refer to Chapter 11, "Compliance")

Figure 10.2

To ensure these accounting functions are being performed properly, management oversight will be needed. In general, this work is typically done by the PSHP's chief financial officer (CFO) or controller, although this will vary by organization. This supervision ensures that all the accounting and general ledger functions are being performed properly and handles any required corrections or adjustments.

Along with managing your past transactions, someone on your PSHP's leadership team must prepare your health plan for its financial future. Typically, it is the CFO who strives to maximize the company's financial position through a variety of financial management tasks like advising the organization's leadership, developing the capital and operating budgets and managing the distribution of profits once your health plan begins recording them. This will determine what percentage of your profits will be reinvested, saved or given to the network providers. This decision also will depend on the business line and state(s) in which you are selling your products because commercial plans have more freedom than government plans for reinvesting any profits.

For example, Texas has an experience rebate provision included in its managed care contracts. So if your organization is selling Medicaid plans in Texas, then you will need to give the state a portion of your net income before taxes because of experience rebate requirements. Keeping all these factors in mind will help the CFO find the best and most intelligent way to use the profits of your business venture.

Analyzing Data

No matter if you are a new or experienced PSHP, in order to successfully guide your organization's ongoing financial management and subsequent plan design decisions, analytics capabilities are essential.

There are different levels of analysis your actuary can perform. The easiest and simplest level is to just follow the general actuarial rules. These rules are basic and look at the hard, obvious facts, like population size and demographics. Say your health plan will serve a population of 2,000 people with an average age of 42 and a gender mix of 30 percent male and 70 percent female. What does this tell an actuary about your population? The honest answer is not much, but the actuary can glean some valuable pieces of information. For example, he or she can advise your organization to tailor your medical management programs toward women and to add benefits targeted at maternity and pediatric services.

With that information, actuaries also can calculate the average member's medical cost. Now, odds are that if the actuary just follows the general actuarial rules, your health plan will do okay — not great, but okay. The main problem is that this level of analysis does not take into account all the other socioeconomic factors that influence healthcare costs.

To more accurately stratify the risk of your member population, many actuaries use a statistical technique called predictive risk modeling. The basic premise is that members' costs as a whole are predictable. By compiling demographic, socioeconomic and clinical data about your entire membership population, an actuary can more accurately set base rates, modify plan designs, adjust care management activities, predict government reimbursement and calculate reserves and RBC.

While this is a more complex evaluation, it will help your actuary read between the lines and better understand the whole population to which you will potentially be selling products. Say your network of providers serves a large geographic area. Parts of this area might be rural, suburban or industrial and each of those locales will impact an attentive actuary's calculations for plan design and financial management.

For example, if your plan insures employees at a suburban convenience store that hires low-income staff, then the actuary can accurately assume several characteristics to be true: the majority of these employees will be overweight and have preexisting conditions that have gone untreated due to their likely financial difficulties. Obviously, these employees will have different health concerns and costs than employees working at a white-collar law firm. Understanding these socioeconomic roots will help to more accurately project costs. For actuaries to really be successful, they have got to get to that level of detail when looking at your entire member population.

Once you get past your first year as a health plan, your actuary's job becomes easier. The overall medical cost of each member will trend somewhat similarly from year to year, so actuaries just need to be aware of changes within your PSHP's member population and the healthcare organizations in your network so they can continuously revise their predictive risk models. In short, they must periodically assess:

- Changes in any of the plan's benefits

- Increases and decreases in provider contract rates

- New medical management policies that will impact utilization

- Removal or addition of risk management strategies

All of these changes can impact cost and, in turn, the actuary's overall calculations for plan design and financial management.

Pricing

In the end, the level playing field that all plans compete on is price. As discussed in Chapter 4, "Plan Design," data and price are all directly linked. An actuary sets the plan's prices using the plan's past performance data, competitors' past performance data, and by monitoring the news to learn about current events and general economic trends or conditions that will likely affect your plan. Price also varies based on various plan characteristics, including network size, wellness programs, free benefits and carve-outs. For example, some plan designs have narrow networks that are paired with reduced out-of-pocket costs. Actuaries combine all of this plan design information with the analyzed population data discussed previously to develop their "magic" formula for the actuarial values assigned to each plan level.

When setting plan prices, it is important for your actuaries to be as close to the bull's eye as possible. Accuracy is your plan's way of making a profit or breaking even, otherwise your plan will lose money. Your price setting can be simple or more complicated depending on the types of products your plan decides to sell.

For example, with commercial products, your PSHP can price plans as aggressively or conservatively as you want, using your actuary's analysis as a guide. But there are consequences associated with both scenarios. Conversely, Medicaid product or plan pricing is relatively straightforward. The government tells you what rates to set and then the actuary's analysis helps identify ways to be more profitable within this rate structure. In essence, your organization is a rate taker, not a rate maker. If your premium prices are too low and very aggressive, then the plan is going to sell a lot of products, but not make a profit. You will be losing money on every life you insure because your claim expenses will be greater than your revenue (for an example, see the case study, *CoOportunity and a Cautionary Tale of Improper Health Plan Pricing*).

On the flip side, if your plan is too conservative and your prices are too high, then the plan is not going to sell a lot of products, but it will — in theory — make a good profit. The danger in this latter scenario is that you will likely lose members to your competitors, and ultimately fail to make money as a business and not fulfill your mission as a healthcare organization.

Case Study
CoOportunity and a Cautionary Tale of Improper Health Plan Pricing

In 2010, in addition to numerous other reforms, the ACA created and funded consumer-operated-and-oriented plans (CO-OPs) as an alternative health insurance option to be offered on public Exchanges and as a means for helping to foster competition in individual marketplaces.

In January 2015, one year after the ACA went into operation, the Iowa Insurance Division (IID) ordered the closure of CoOportunity, one of 23 nonprofit CO-OP insurance companies. Specifically IID commandeered CoOportunity, which enrolled about 100,000 individual and group members in Iowa and Nebraska, because steep losses were overwhelming the plan. Premium revenue was insufficient to cover enrollees' high use of medical services and the Centers for Medicare & Medicaid Services (CMS) denied any extra funding. While the Iowa situation was unfortunate, it offers lessons for newly formed health plans:

- If plan prices are set too low and a member population is sicker and uses more services than originally anticipated, members' premiums cannot fully cover their medical expenses even though the plan may be rapidly increasing its total enrollment

- Risk-Based Capital (RBC) reserves need to be fully capitalized if not over capitalized to help account for premiums gaps when the health risk profiles and utilization patterns of a potential health plan-covered population are unknown

Despite the IID's story, many industry observers believe "CO-OPs have 'injected welcome measures of choice and competition into the health insurance marketplace' and in [year two] have already overcome a lot of their financial pitfalls," according to a January 2015 article published in the "Journal of the American Medical Association" (JAMA).

Dr. Eli Adashi, former Dean of Medicine and Biological Sciences at Brown University and co-author of the JAMA article, said in an interview that it is not easy for startups like CO-OPs to compete with "the giants that are currently ruling the market." They are operating under tight budgets, and when something goes awry, "there aren't all that many options for them in terms of course correction."

But the future of CO-OPs remains "promising if uncertain," Dr. Adashi argued, because they have, at the very least, encouraged more competitive pricing in the exchanges.

"The market will determine whether or not they have the right stuff," Adashi said. "We do think the potential is still there."

Source: Valence Health summary of JAMA,
"Modern Healthcare" and "New York Times" articles

How you price your plans is up to you, but keep in mind that your rates are locked in place for a year, so you do not have the opportunity to pivot up or down. You also need to remember that the recent shifts in the industry are making pricing increasingly transparent to all — both the purchaser and deliverer of healthcare services can more easily identify the cost of services. This trend will likely only continue in the years to come and should be present in the all of your plan's pricing decisions (for more information on plan transparency, refer to Chapter 4, "Plan Design").

Tracking Key Health Plan Actuarial Considerations and Financial Management Metrics

Performing regular data analysis can help your PSHP maximize its return on investment and identify both early warning signs of trouble and indicators of success. By tracking key inputs and outputs, you can continually enhance your health plan so it retains members, remains financially stable and earns high patient satisfaction scores. Below are key actuarial considerations and financial management metrics that should be measured continuously:

- Plan's insurance risk
- Risk management strategies
- Potential member population size
- Actual member enrollment
- Enrollee demographics
- Enrollee medical conditions
- Enrollee treatment information
- Enrollee healthcare costs
- Government reimbursement rates and policies
- Plan reserves
- Plan capital
- Plan equity
- Risk-based capital
- Plan taxes

- Accounts payable
- Accounts receivable
- Plan rates
- Plan designs
- Plan incentives
- Wellness programs
- Free benefits
- Carve-outs
- Medical management services
- Operating budgets and variance to date
- Provider contract rates
- Network size
- Plan profits
- Employee payroll

Industry Terminology Related to Actuarial Considerations and Financial Management

Asset Risk   Risk related to market changes or poor investment performance of a financial asset (e.g., shares, options, futures or currency).

Source: RiskyThinking.com

Authorized Control Level Risk-Based Capital   Theoretical amount of capital plus surplus an insurance company should maintain.

Source: National Association of Insurance Commissioners

Business Risk   The probability of loss inherent in an organization's operations and environment (such as competition and adverse economic conditions) that may impair its ability to provide returns on investment. Business risk plus the financial risk arising from use of debt (borrowed capital and/or trade credit) equal total corporate risk.

Source: BusinessDictionary.com

Capital Wealth in the form of money or assets, taken as a sign of the financial strength of an individual, organization or nation, and assumed to be available for development or investment.

Source: BusinessDictionary.com

Carve-Outs Health insurance carve-outs concern a method to separate specific services from general healthcare contracts. A different contract and payment arrangement covers the designated "carved-out" services. Carve-outs also include services or benefits provided to a smaller segment of an employee population, or used to offer additional benefits under a different insurance carrier.

Source: eHow.com

Credit Risk Probability of loss from a debtor's default. In banking, credit risk is a major factor in determination of interest rate on a loan; the longer the term of the loan, usually the higher the interest rate.

Source: BusinessDictionary.com

Electronic Medical Record A real-time patient health record with access to evidence-based decision support tools that can be used to aid clinicians in decision making. The EMR can automate and streamline a clinician's work-flow, ensuring that all clinical information is communicated. It can also prevent delays in response that result in gaps in care. The EMR can also support the collection of data for uses other than clinical care, such as billing, quality management, outcome reporting and public health disease surveillance and reporting. Synonymous with Electronic Health Record or EHR.

Source: Office of the National Coordinator for Health IT

Equity Net worth of a person or company computed by subtracting total liabilities from the total assets.

Source: BusinessDictionary.com

Health Information Exchange (HIE) The electronic movement of health-related information among organizations according to nationally recognized standards. The goal of health information exchange is to facilitate access to and retrieval of clinical data to provide safer, timelier, efficient, effective, equitable and patient-centered care.

Source: U.S. Department of Health and Human Services

Practice Management Systems A tool or type of software to help manage day-to-day operations in physicians' offices. These systems are often used for financial and administrative functions, and can also be linked with a patient's health or dental record. Practice management software can help track billing and demographic data, along with appointment scheduling.

Source: U.S. Department of Health and Human Services

Reserve   The amount kept by the insurer to be able to cover all of the company's debts. This term also can refer to an amount earmarked by the insurer for a specific purpose.

Source: Valence Health

Risk-Based Capital (RBC)   Money that must be retained by a savings institution to leverage the risks associated with conducting day-to-day business. Risk-based capital requirements were enacted in 1989 and require the saving institution to have more money on hand for higher risk assets.

Source: BusinessDictionary.com

Underwriting Risk   The probability that an actual return on an investment will be lower than the expected return.

Source: BusinessDictionary.com

Chapter Eleven
Compliance

To legally drive a bus, there are certain traffic laws you must follow and registration and auto insurance coverage requirements you must be able to prove — for both the bus itself and its driver. You can always take a risk and drive for a little while with an expired driver's license or outdated registration, but soon enough you will get caught and have to face the consequences.

The same is true for your provider-sponsored health plan (PSHP). It has insurance and payor ground rules and regulations to which you must comply. As a health plan, your PSHP will be bound by state insurance and product laws. If you have public exchange, Medicare and/or Medicaid products, you also will have to keep abreast of federal and state rules and regulations. This requires ongoing monitoring as new laws and administrative rules are continuously being passed, issued or updated. While you can always go above and beyond these baselines requirements to distinguish your health plan from competitors, you cannot fall below (see the *Driscoll Health Plan* case study at the end of this chapter).

In short, your compliance department keeps your PSHP in line before the regulatory entities do. This team is charged with monitoring rules and laws and is responsible for:

- Identifying and managing regulation violations

- Preventing future violations from occurring

- Developing and implementing controls to resolve current violations

- Monitoring the effectiveness of these new controls

- Advising the plan on existing controls and how to comply with new rules
  and regulations

Clearly, your compliance team should be intimately familiar with the regulations you will be working under, as well as requirements specifically related to selling commercial, Medicare and/or Medicaid products before your PSHP can serve its members. This knowledge will help compliance staff initially set up the PSHP and secure any necessary state approvals. This effort includes everything from filling out the initial registration documents for designing and implementing the required programs.

> ### Expert Insight
>
> *"During a PSHP's development process, providers sometimes make the mistake of acting like a provider rather than like a health plan. This is because they often don't have an accurate sense of the scope of what is involved when becoming a health plan. Being a health plan goes far beyond being a provider organization.*
>
> *Compliance forces you to take a closer look at this since you're responsible for a larger scale now. You're no longer just responsible for the clinical needs, but also for paying claims. You must recognize that even though you may start as a provider group, you will ultimately grow to be a different kind of organization and you have to take responsibility for that.*
>
> *You are entering a different industry when you develop a health plan, which means that there will be totally new responsibilities, expectations and more new rules than you could have imagined."*
>
> **– R. Todd Stockard**
> President and Co-Founder, Valence Health

Therefore, to help best inform your build, buy or partner/outsource decisions related to PSHP compliance, we have devoted the rest of this chapter to explaining four key components that will assure your PSHP abides by the relevant rules and interacts with the appropriate regulatory entities.

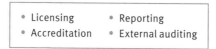

Essential Health Plan Compliance Needs

Source: Valence Health

• Licensing	• Reporting
• Accreditation	• External auditing

Figure 11.1

Licensing

In general, compliant PSHPs need to attain all applicable licenses prior to starting operations. As mentioned in the chapter introduction, the types of licenses required vary dramatically depending on state regulations, product type, contract requirements and local marketplace competition. This means that a preferred provider organization in rural Nebraska will probably require different licenses than a health maintenance organization operating in urban New York City. They also will have different requirements for attaining these licenses — such as the capital reserve requirements (refer to Chapter 10, "Actuarial Considerations and Financial Management," for more information).

Before your health plan can begin operating, you need to determine exactly what licenses your state agencies' internal departments and/or the National Association of Insurance Commissions (NAIC) require for your organization, and what licenses the applicable professional boards require for your individual providers or PSHP employees. While the names vary, each state has a regulatory body or agency that grants professional licenses to various organizations and individual professions. For example, case managers may need to have state and federal certifications in one state and no certifications in a neighboring state.

Despite these differences, the central reason for requiring licenses is the same across all states and entities: to make sure all health plans agree to operate and conduct business in compliance with state and/or national laws and regulations, and to protect the best interests of their citizens.

Common Health Plan Licenses/Requirements

Source: Valence Health

- Uniform Certificate of Authority Application (UCAA)
- Third-Party Administrator (TPA) License
- Utilization Review Agent (URA) License
- Individual Employee Licenses

Figure 11.2

Some common health plan licenses include:

- **Uniform Certificate of Authority Application (UCAA)**
  The UCAA is a uniform application through NAIC that allows the Chief Executive Officer (CEO) or Chief Operating Officer (COO) of your health plan to apply for an insurance license in almost any state. Most states still require additional requirements above and beyond this baseline application, but nevertheless, having your UCAA helps streamline the process for obtaining licenses in other states.

- **Third-Party Administrator (TPA)**

  If your health plan is partnering with a TPA to help with some of its insurance functions, like claims administration and management, then it is probable that your partner will need a TPA license before it can conduct business in your state (for more information on using TPAs or vendors, refer to Chapter 3, "Determining Your PSHP's Comprehensive Execution Strategy"). While it is the vendor's job to obtain this license, your organization needs to ensure that your partner has the TPA license before it performs services for your health plan.

- **Utilization Review Agent (URA)**

  Certain states require a URA license to address the specific ways in which your PSHP will handle its medical management activities and its appeal processes. This application is typically available on your state's Department of Insurance website along with details about any applicable fees, additional documentation requirements and possible discounts. If you outsource all of your utilization management services, then your partner will need this license on your behalf. This license is typically renewed every two years, and in some states, this simply involves paying a renewal fee. In other markets, it requires fingerprint screenings, background checks and biographical affidavits from various members of your organization.

- **Employee Licenses**

  If you have any physicians, nurses, social workers, medical directors or community health workers on your PSHP's staff or in your affiliated healthcare organization, your state may require them all to have valid individual licenses. Your health plan is required to have properly credentialed employees or partners, so organizations typically conduct annual reviews to identify expired licenses or new limitations that need to be addressed.

Expert Insight

"Most states and accreditation organizations require health plans to have policies and procedures in place to annually review the licensures of its employees. This helps ensure the licenses have not expired and that no adverse action, limitation or restriction has been placed on the licenses. For physicians, this can be done by checking the state medical board and national specialty certifications, while the licenses for nurses and other allied health professionals can be verified on the state nursing board, Nursys® and other professional boards/certifications."

– Stephanie Holland
Manager of Regulatory Compliance and Quality, Valence Health

Accreditation

After your PSHP attains the necessary licenses, you may choose to evaluate becoming an accredited organization. Almost every health plan wants this accreditation — it is just a standard of business. This achievement proves your health plan is satisfying nationally recognized, evidence-based guidelines for quality services.

Accreditation also can help differentiate your plan from competitors and allow you to enter into contracts that require this higher standard. Think of it this way: if you are choosing between a bus that has the National Transportation Advisory Board's Best Maintenance Award displayed on its door and one that does not, which vehicle would you choose to ride?

In addition, health plans that want to sell products on a public exchange must be accredited by the National Committee for Quality Assurance (NCQA) or Utilization Review Accreditation Commission (URAC), which are the two accrediting bodies approved by the U.S. Department of Health and Human Services (HHS).

Selecting Your Accrediting Body:
NCQA versus URAC

NCQA and URAC are two well-respected accrediting bodies commonly used by health plans. Since price is comparable for the two, health plans often select one over the other based on what is preferred locally or what your staff has previous experience with. Below are several other key characteristics your PSHP may consider when making its decision:

NCQA:

* Recognized as the national leader in accreditation since it has accredited more health plans

* Offers more resources for assistance

* Established in the market longer for comprehensive accreditation

URAC:

* Required for some state utilization management (UM) licensures and well-respected by regulators

* Established in the market longer for focused UM certifications

Both:

* Provide comprehensive health plan accreditation as well as a myriad of focused certifications, including UM, case management, disease management and accountable care organizations (ACOs)

* Accepted equally by most state and federal exchanges

Source: Valence Health

However, not all health plans choose to become accredited. For example, most states do not require Medicaid plans to attain accreditation, and many small local or regional plans do not have outside pressure in their geographic region to pursue this option or are deterred by the cost.

If your PSHP chooses to pursue accreditation while you are still designing your plan, you can pursue a provisional or interim accreditation through the NCQA or URAC. During this time, the entity will review your preliminary policies and procedures to see if they will satisfy their standards for each service.

Typically, it takes a health plan 18 months to prepare for its first NCQA and URAC accreditation. This initial process involves a team effort to ensure your PSHP and any of your vendor partners are meeting requirements. The accreditation entities themselves are a helpful resource during this time. For example, NCQA provides seminars, publications and technical support if your team needs more guidance. Once your health plan has enrolled more members, then the accrediting entity will review additional information to determine your plan's accreditation status.

Both NCQA and URAC also require ongoing re-accreditation. Although these processes differ slightly between the two, they both include quality measures, a Consumer Assessment of Healthcare Providers and Systems (CAHPS) aspect, and on-site and off-site evaluations. The results of these evaluations, which occur on an annual or triennial basis, will determine your health plan's accreditation status. To prepare for any re-accreditations, your PSHP team will need to again monitor any new regulations and resolve any past violations or warnings.

Reporting and External Audits

Even if your health plan obtains all the necessary licenses and becomes accredited, several state and federal agencies will need to continuously track your plan's business operations, market conduct and financial performance indicators to see if you are complying with their mandates and are financially stable. Other public agencies typically do this by requiring periodic reports and external audits, which are publicly accessible.

The rules surrounding these reports and external audits vary drastically, depending upon your product line, distribution model and states where you operate. While the frequency, required information and logistics needed for reports and audits will change depending upon your specific situation, one thing is true for all health plans: you need to take these activities seriously to ensure compliance and avoid penalties, fines or lack of payment.

> ### Expert Insight
>
> *"There are multiple agencies a health plan must report to depending upon its unique situation. At Security Health Plan, we submit reports to both the NAIC and our Wisconsin Office of the Commissioner of Insurance. We also have a Medicare Advantage product and Exchange product that report to the Centers for Medicare & Medicaid Service (CMS) along with a Medicaid product that is affiliated with our state's Department of Health Services."*
>
> **– Geri Batten, CPA and CMA**
> Controller, Security Health Plan

As a new PSHP, you may receive a heightened level of scrutiny from state and federal entities regarding the financial relationship between your providers and the parent company to ensure all transactions between the different entities are ethical and do not violate any insurance principles (because some of your providers will be providing care and also receiving premiums).

Due to the highly variable nature of the insurance industry and increased scrutiny of PSHPs, many health plans rely on a General Counsel, Chief Financial Officer (CFO) or Controller to advise them on regulatory reporting and external audits requirements. When Valence Health works with clients in these areas, we traditionally suggest dividing the work, with the CFO or Controller focusing on the financial performance indicators (such as financial statements and transactions with affiliated companies), while the General Counsel focuses on market conduct performance indicators (which include clinical quality metrics, evaluation of sales and marketing practices, analysis of complaints and grievances, etc.). For more information on CFOs' and Controllers' roles within a PSHP, refer to Chapter 10, "Actuarial Considerations and Financial Management." This logical division not only makes the work surrounding reporting and external audits more manageable, but also mirrors the structure of most regulatory agencies.

These members of your staff will review your plan's products, target membership, geographic footprint and method of plan distribution and use this information as road signs to direct them toward the correct regulatory agencies and their applicable statutes, administrative codes, and guidance or bulletins, which are available online.

In general, statutes are laws that were passed by the legislature. Each statute will have a corresponding administrative code, which contains details that the corresponding regulating agency wrote about the statute. For example, maybe the legislature passes a statute that requires Wisconsin to create an independent review organization that can function as the ultimate determiner for disputes about experimental care. In response, the regulating agency will develop a new portion of its administrative code to determine things like if there will be a certification process, etc. Further additions or amendments to this administrative code are published in guidances or bulletins.

This process and the general categories for the statutes are similar across the nation, but the administrative codes will vary and change over time. For this reason, it is important to stay abreast of changing conditions and new requirements. Without this diligent effort to maintain compliance, your health plan may inadvertently violate new regulations, resulting in a variety of consequences.

You must also create and then update your database of regulatory reporting, external auditing and statute requirements to maintain compliance. These changes must then be communicated to the appropriate staff.

As your staff navigates new rules or regulations and tries to remain compliant with old ones, most regulatory agencies are willing and eager to provide assistance. The relationship between your health plan and the regulatory agencies is built on mutual respect as both parties strive to increase the plan's quality and mitigate its risks. For this reason, regulatory agencies frequently provide guidance and will work with health plans to both follow and improve regulations.

Expert Insight

"Developing a PSHP has been such an incredible journey and having relationships at the regulatory level — both from a state and federal perspective — has been critical.

Insurance is a fairly regulated business, so we see a real need to have open, positive dialogue with the State Commissioner or Director of Insurance in your state. We think the world of our respective departments, and they have been remarkable in helping us navigate a complicated process."

– Jason Montrie
President, Land of Lincoln Health

For example, say there is a new type of Medicaid plan in Illinois and neither the health plans nor the state knows how it will work. There will be a lot of communication between the plans and state. Maybe the plans believe a requirement is not practical, so the state will decide to extend the timeline for completing the task. In this situation, both entities work together to achieve the most desirable outcomes. This positive relationship extends beyond the initial implementation to include continued guidance. As issues continue to arise, your plan can always turn to the agency or offer up its own suggestions.

Internal Audits

While external audits are a critical way for state and federal agencies to monitor your plan's compliance, it does not end there. You also will have to take on the responsibility for conducting internal audits of your plan to proactively identify and fix issues before they result in violations. These internal audits and data analytics also drive continuous process improvements.

> **Expert Insight**
>
> *"Ongoing compliance work involves a lot of auditing to find out what you don't know. Once you have identified a problem, you need to figure out how to fix it, implement the change and then do another audit to see if your new controls are working. Bottom line, you're always working on compliance in a health plan."*
>
> **– Allison Hoffman**
> Manager of Quality Management Program, Valence Health

Your internal audits can, and should, be performed on almost any health plan function that can be measured and quantified. At a minimum, this includes:

- Provider credentialing
- Claims processing
- Enrollment and eligibility processes
- Network standards regarding accessibility and availability
- Member- or provider-facing programs

More information on credentialing and provider networks can be found in Chapter 6, "Network Development and Management," while additional details on claims processing and enrollment and eligibility processes is located in Chapter 9, "Claims Administration and Management."

Performing regular audits will keep PSHP staff focused on consistently following established policies and processes. It also helps leadership gauge the effectiveness of these current initiatives against internal or external benchmarks and identify processes or people who are not meeting the desired standards. From this information, your health plan can overcome barriers by implementing corrective actions, ranging from new policies to additional employee education. Future internal audits can then assess the effectiveness of these improvements and foster the creation of additional initiatives.

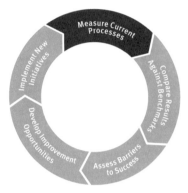

Internal Audit Process for Continuous Process Improvements

Source: Valence Health

Figure 11.3

It is important to know that if your plan is ever found to be noncompliant, the consequences will vary depending on the severity of the violation. The primary consequences of violating a regulation include a corrective action plan, financial penalties and suspension or loss of licensure.

- **Corrective Action Plan**
  The least-severe consequence for a health plan is a corrective action plan. For example, imagine CMS, during its triennial review, informing your organization that it is required to submit an expense report on a quarterly basis. Due to simple human error, your staff thought this report was due annually. It is a simple, perhaps even common mistake, but now your staff must draft and complete a corrective action plan. In short, this plan identifies the problem, outlines how you will fix it and sets a timeline for next steps. CMS will then review your corrective action plan and adjust it as needed.

- **Financial Penalties**
  Other common consequences are fines, sanctions or forfeitures. These financial penalties can range from $500 to hundreds of thousands of dollars and are delineated in federal or state law, statute or code. For example, if you do not meet state or federal clean claim laws, then there are assigned penalties that your state's regulatory agency can enforce.

- **Suspension or Loss of Licensure**
  The most severe consequence your health plan can receive is a suspension or loss of licensure. When a plan's license is suspended, it can still retain its current member-

ship, but cannot sell products to new members until the violation is resolved. For severe violations, like fraud and abuse, a health plan could potentially lose its license and be shut down.

 The PSHPs we have worked with over the years have all been deeply committed to quality and operational integrity. In fact, they go out of their way to assure everything they build and maintain within their operation infrastructures is both highly efficient and always in compliance."

– Lori Fox Ward, RN, BSN
Senior Vice President of Market Solutions, Valence Health

To avoid these consequences, internal audits and data analytics should be conducted and examined periodically to enhance internal processes and proactively prepare for external audits. This can even allow your plan to begin resolving any issues with an internal corrective action plan before the regulatory agency learns about them. It is far better to show the agency your month-old audit with its corresponding internal corrective action plan and preliminary improvements than to let the agency find your problems for you. This not only makes fixing the problem easier, but also can reduce any consequences. ⬯

Case Study:
Going Well Beyond the Required Case Management Compliance Guidelines – *Driscoll Health Plan*

The Driscoll Health Plan (DHP) is a provider-sponsored health plan that serves more than 140,000 members and is the dominant Medicaid health plan in south Texas. As the primary driver of population health management in its service area, DHP has launched a number of clinical quality initiatives that far exceed what its plan is required to provide to be compliant with Texas' Medicaid guidelines.

DHP established the Cadena de Madres program to provide prenatal education, lactation consulting and nutritional counseling to pregnant women enrolled in the State of Texas Access Reform program. Its approach was to:

- Gather data and develop and distribute "report cards" to address obstetrics (OB) outcomes

- Hold meetings to share data and educate OB leaders in the community

- Develop incentives for high-performing OB providers, members and hospitals

- Hold hospital meetings regarding OB and neonatal intensive care unit (NICU) guidelines

- Financially support the recruitment of maternal fetal medicine specialists
- Develop a neonate transfer policy for the plan's infants

Results:

- Hosted more than 1,380 showers in 49 locations with 8,300 attendees
- Dramatically reduced NICU days and average length of stay since program's inception
- Increased vaginal births and reduced cesarean sections
- Reduced the region's preterm births by 34% (one of the clinical conditions that carry the highest costs and can lead to lifelong health problems)

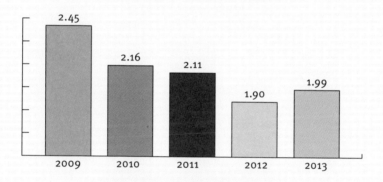

NICU Days Per Delivery
Source: Mary Peterson, MD, MSHCA, FACHE

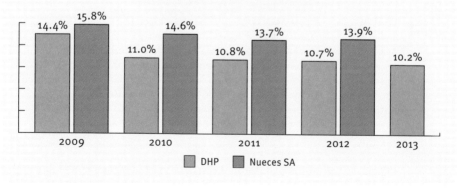

Preterm Births (<37 Weeks)
Source: Mary Peterson, MD, MSHCA, FACHE

Tracking Key Health Plan Compliance Metrics

Performing regular data analysis can help your PSHP maximize its return on investment and identify both early warning signs of trouble and indicators of success. By tracking key inputs and outputs, you can continually enhance your health plan so it retains members, remains financially stable and earns high patient satisfaction scores. Below are key compliance metrics that should be measured continuously:

- Applicable organizational licensing requirements for states your plan serves
- Applicable individual licensing requirements
- State and/or federal licensing regulations by product type
- Network and payor contract requirements for licensure
- Local marketplace licensure and ac-creditation status for competitive plans
- Prior staff and leadership experience with accreditation
- State insurance license requirements beyond the UCAA
- Proof of TPA or vendor licenses
- State URA license requirements
- Plan's credentialing standards
- Re-accreditation requirements
- Plan's accreditation status (if accreditation is pursued)
- Plan's market conduct performance indicators
- Plan's financial performance indicators

- Reporting and external audit rules and requirements
- Applicable monitoring of statutes, administrative codes, and guidance or bulletins
- Communication standards and timelines regarding new regulatory rules and requirements
- Policies and processes for conducting internal audits and compliance activities
- Number of violations identified via external and internal audits
- Number of violations fixed by new initiatives
- Number of violations unresolved after new initiatives
- Severity of violations
- Number of consequences from external agencies for violations
- Type of consequences from external agencies for violations
- Remediation plans and remediation progress tracking and reporting procedures

Industry Terminology Related to Compliance

Accreditation   Process in which a state or other standard-setting regulatory organization determines whether an entity seeking to provide services subject to that organization's authority meets acceptable standards for such purposes. For example, commercial insurers domiciled in a state that passes all the National Association of Insurance Commissioners (NAIC) model acts and other-wise passes muster will be acceptable security in other states.

Source: National Association of Insurance Commissioners

Claim   A request for payment that you or your healthcare provider submits to your health insurer when you get items or services you think are covered.

Source: Healthcare.gov

License   Certification of appropriate authority issued by a regulatory body to allow an entity to operate as an insurer or an insurance agent after certain standards have been met.

Source: International Risk Management Institute

National Association of Insurance Commissioners (NAIC)   The U.S. standard-setting and regulatory support organization created and governed by the chief insurance regulators from the 50 states, the District of Columbia and five U.S. territories. Through the NAIC, state insurance regulators establish standards and best practices, conduct peer review and coordinate their regulatory oversight.

Source: NAIC

Third-Party Administrator (TPA)   A person or organization that processes claims and performs other administrative services in accordance with a service contract, usually in the field of employee benefits. More specifically, a TPA is neither the insurer (provider) nor the insured (employees or plan participants), but handles the administration of the plan including processing, adjudication, and negotiation of claims, recordkeeping and maintenance of the plan.

Source: MyCafeteriaPlan.com

Uniform Certificate of Authority Application (UCAA)   A process designed to allow insurers to file copies of the same application for admission in numerous states. Each state that accepts the UCAA is designated as a uniform state. While each uniform state still performs its own independent review of each application, the need to file different applications, in different formats, has been eliminated for all states that accept the uniform application.

Source: National Association of Insurance Commissioners

Utilization Management   The evaluation of the medical necessity, appropriateness and efficiency of the use of healthcare services, procedures and facilities under the provisions of the applicable health benefits plan, sometimes called "utilization review."

Source: Utilization Review Accreditation Commission

Utilization Review Accreditation Commission (URAC)   An independent, non-profit organization, URAC is a well-known leader in promoting healthcare quality through its accreditation, education and measurement programs.

Source: URAC.org

Utilization Review Agent (URA)   People working on behalf of a health insurance company who review a request for medical treatment and confirm a health plan provides coverage for medical services. This helps the company minimize costs and determine if the recommended treatment is appropriate.

Source: Health.HowStuffWorks.com

Chapter Twelve
Health Plan Technology

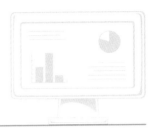

One key component that will impact every area of your provider-sponsored health plan (PSHP) is technology. As the entire U.S. healthcare industry continues to move toward value-based reimbursement, it is critical that payors and providers adopt technology that supports outcomes-based reimbursement models. As mentioned in Chapter 2, "How Today's PSHPs are Different," actively using these technologies and the data that fuel them is one of the key differences that will make your PSHP much more successful than what some unsuccessful health plans experienced in the 1990s.

> ### Expert Insight
> *"Value-based delivery of care is fast becoming a mandate in the healthcare industry. This is enabled by an emerging real-time, interoperable technological architecture and framework. Healthcare payors and administrators need a future-proof technological framework that offers the flexibility and control to handle their needs, both today and tomorrow. Selection and implementation of a technical architecture that is service-oriented and standards-based allows the health plan to incrementally add new business services without the labor and potential cost of upgrading other key operating business functions."*
>
> **– Suzanne Engels**
> Vice President of Professional Services, Aldera

By accessing or developing transparent and connected technological capabilities, your PSHP and your provider network have the potential to more effectively collaborate. Imagine if both your health plan and provider network had the same holistic, real-time view of members'/patients' health history, medical treatment, benefits package, other in-network providers, etc. Fortunately, this type of interconnectivity is now a reality, and there are countless examples of how population health management technology is helping encourage payor-provider collaboration, reduce administrative hassles and costs and improve health outcomes.

From our own firsthand experience, Valence Health's clients use our technologies and others to specifically align payor and provider interactions around things like setting preventative care priorities, closing care gaps and assuring post-acute care follow-up in order to prevent future readmissions. If your PSHP would like to do the same, it will need all available data.

In an ideal world, your PSHP's essential population health management-enabling technologies should connect all of your providers with any health information exchanges (HIEs) in your community. More and more geographic areas are developing these exchanges to facilitate the sharing of healthcare data and information electronically among organizations in a region or community to help provide a holistic view of a patients'/members' clinical history.

> **Expert Insight**
>
> *"In the future, health plans will need to be able to interact with a Health Information Exchange. This will allow them to gather the necessary clinical data or supply the financial data that is needed to manage an individual's healthcare from end to end."*
>
> **– Daniel Knies**
> Chief Technology Officer, Aldera

To effectively communicate with HIEs, you will need enterprise solutions that are based on open-exchange technology architecture and frameworks. These frameworks support interoperability for easier integration with things likes clinical systems, HIEs, private and public health insurance marketplaces and electronic health records (EHRs).

Appropriately using these collaborative technologies will clearly impact all of your plan's technology architecture, software and hardware procurement and maintenance decisions. Therefore, before making your technology related execution strategy decisions, it is important to ensure your team has explored its build, buy or partner/outsource options to source the technologies and supporting skill sets related to your PSHP's population health management needs and objectives (for more information on execution strategy, refer to Chapter 3, "Determining Your PSHP's Comprehensive Execution Strategy").

No matter how your PSHP selects and rolls out any technologies and decision support systems, Valence Health believes that five technologies will be core to your plan's success (see Figure 12.1).

Externally Facing* Health Plan Technology Solutions	Internally Facing ** Health Plan Technology Solutions
• Population health and care management technology solutions • Internet portal technologies * *Interface with or can be accessed by plan members or its network providers*	• Claims processing platform • Call center technologies • Business intelligence or analytic tools **Largely support the internal operations and/ or business needs of your plan's executive team and owners*

Source: Valence Health
Figure 12.1

Population Health and Care Management Technology Solutions

With the help of data mining software, population health management solutions often acquire data from disparate practice management systems and EHR systems. This clinical information can then be augmented with payor claims, hospital admissions discharge and transfer (ADTs) data, lab data, pharmacy data, health risk assessment (HRA) data and more to present a comprehensive view of all services rendered to patients in a community, the members of your PSHP and the healthcare providers.

Comparing this data to accepted evidence-based guidelines, your plan's in-network physicians can see which of their patients have care gaps or how they are performing with respect to clinical guidelines, benchmarks and incentive programs they agreed to in your contracting process.

For health plan executives who use population health technology, users can track and monitor the quality performance of individual providers and provider organizations through specialty profiles, primary care physician profiles, etc. In most population health technology solutions, administrative users then have the ability to compare these quality metrics to network benchmarks or industry standards, like the Health Effectiveness Data and Information Set, National Quality Forum, Physician Quality Reporting System or other specialty associations. This allows health plans to assess barriers and develop improvement opportunities to achieve better outcomes and promote greater consistency among its providers.

In concert with these larger population health objectives, case management systems can effectively provide medical management services in ways that assure the entire care team is kept abreast of a member's progress (see Figure 12.2 for an example). In a health plan environment, care management technology needs to address three core functions: utilization management (UM), case management (CM), and disease management (DM).

Case management technologies should be designed to make everyone's lives easier. While some of these systems provide UM, CM and DM separately, others provide them across one integrated platform. Regardless of the chosen structure, impactful technology will create an integrated member record that is logically embedded into your plan's case managers' workflow, thus also improving productivity (see Figure 12.2).

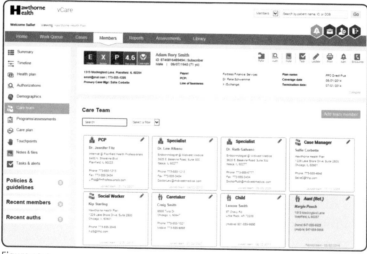

Valence Health's vCare© Technology Offers a Unified Member View

Source: Valence Health

Figure 12.2

The care management technology should enable UM, CM and DM operations and assure resulting data and information that comes from these efforts to be integrated with other population health information to provide a comprehensive view of PSHP members' needs and services being delivered to them. This can help improve patient outcomes while lowering healthcare costs. Other benefits of integrating case management technology are outlined in Figure 12.3.

CM staff can use either your plan's care management technology or interface with your business intelligence tools (discussed in another section of this chapter) to help identify high-risk beneficiaries, or members who might benefit from CM or DM activities, like end-of-life planning (see the case study, *Improving End-of-Life Care for Medicare Advantage Members*). Whether your plan uses one system or an interface between two technologies, risk stratification and/or predictive modeling algorithms will separate the plan's members into various risk groups. The output is a registry of members with chronic conditions and their assigned risk scores, which are used to target segments of the population who can be impacted the most with preventative care and chronic disease management.

Benefits of Integrating Care Management Technology with the EHR and/or Claims Processing System

- Allows users to view a member's demographics, benefit plan, primary care physician, eligibility, payor information and claims history
- Helps identify the medical cost and utilization drivers
- Facilitates collaboration between health plan and healthcare staff to more effectively coordinate and manage medical management activities
- Allows physicians and their office staff to see case plans and any completed CM activities or concerns
- Facilitates member referrals between UM, CM and DM, while reducing unnecessary repetition of basic member information
- Helps attract high-quality providers to your network by giving them user-friendly systems to work with

Source: Valence Health
Figure 12.3

To more specifically support your plan's UM needs, your care management technology should help determine if members' hospital admissions are medically necessary. To facilitate this decision-making process, relevant guidelines can be embedded within your care management technology. These guidelines and corresponding medical policies can be national, state-specific or unique to your health plan.

These guidelines also can trigger other process requirements around turnaround times, prior authorization lists, denial reason codes and communication rules for items like authorization or denial letters/communications. Since these requirements help objectively determine if claims and services will or will not be paid, care management technology often can be used to send notices and deadlines to other functional areas in your health plan that then will have to complete these other activities.

Depending upon the care management technology being used, these authorizations also can be securely transferred from physicians to your health plan by a variety of methods. Some systems also contain authorization auto-approval logic. This feature can save significant time by immediately approving certain authorizations. Over time, health plans can use their data from previous authorizations to determine which services still need or do not need to be subjected to your plan's prior authorization processes.

Case Study:

Improving End-of-Life Care for Medicare Advantage Members – *Gundersen Health Plan*

The Gundersen Health Plan, part of the Gundersen Health System, covers 80,000 members in Wisconsin and Iowa and offers a five-star-rated Medicare Advantage plan called Senior Preferred. The Gundersen Health System is an international pioneer in end-of-life planning that reduces unwanted treatment, enhances dignity and saves money.

Respecting Choices®: A Model of Advance Care Planning (RC) was started in 1991 in an effort to reinvent advance care planning for individuals in the last two years of life. Traditionally, clinicians gave patients a brochure about advance directives and asked a cursory question about their plans. Not surprisingly, this approach worked poorly. After studying the problem, Gundersen's leaders recommended a system redesign such that:

- Advance care planning is built into all routine patient care

- It is based on in-depth, high-quality conversations that are skillfully facilitated by trained professionals

- The conversations result in a clear plan

- The plan is available wherever the patient receives care

- The plan is interpreted with thoughtful medical judgment when the patient cannot advocate for himself or herself

- The healthcare system offers a range of services in multiple settings to honor the care plan

Adopting this approach, Gundersen Health System has reduced unwanted hospitalizations, reduced the cost of care and decreased the intensity of hospital care in the last six months of its patients' lives. All told, for every $1 spent on advance care planning reduces the cost of healthcare by $2.

Source: "Return on Investment: Implementation of Respecting Choices® Model of Advance Care Planning," GundersenHealth.org

CM activities also should be supported by care management technology that supports simple and more complex medical and behavioral case management. These CM services strive to engage members in self-directed care by helping them return to and maintain their optimal level of health and well-being through ongoing assessments, interventions and facilitation techniques. Members and their corresponding stratified risk scores, which represent expected future costs, will be pre-identified frequently by your technology and then staff can confirm which patients qualify for CM.

Some case management technology systems even contain embedded algorithmic assessments or links to national, state-specific or organization-specific care guidelines and criteria that staff can use to generate recommended care plans. Oftentimes, staff also can use the system to conduct a quality-of-life assessment, track patient interventions and monitor progress toward healthcare goals.

Your plan's DM programs also can be supported by care management technology solutions. Here, your software will generally identify plan members who meet the criteria for a disease management program for certain chronic conditions like diabetes, asthma, etc. These members can be routed automatically to the applicable DM services using customized system triggers. Outreach initiatives in these programs also are frequently supported by technological solutions. Even the seemingly manual task of sending mailings can be scheduled within your systems so that staff is notified automatically when program materials should be sent.

Many organizations also are integrating telehealth into their care management arsenal by delivering disease management information through a variety of methods. For example, Interactive Voice Response (IVR) systems gather health data from members through a series of prompts and deliver computer-generated feedback on DM topics.

Another form of telehealth being integrated into care management is personal medical devices. These provide patients with portable technology that can remotely monitor things like vital signs and symptoms. Thermometers, pedometers, glucose meters, scales and body composite analyzers are just a few of the many devices that can capture patients' health information at home or on the go. The data collected by these devices can then be recorded manually by the patient or automatically be directed back to providers, case managers or both. Some technologies even allow the data to be added to EHRs.

Case Study:
vCare's© Approach to Case Management

vCare is Valence Health's care management technology solution that integrates key patient-focused functionality to better coordinate care and achieve population management goals. It automates case management referrals, care coordination and outreach to ensure that everyone on a patient's care team has the same information.

vCare's workflow applications allow case managers to generate individualized care plans for case management candidates. Case managers can document, track and facilitate care plans and community resource participation as part of their daily workflow. vCare can be used by your own care coordinators or Valence Health's care management staff to provide outreach, assessment and a wide variety of case management services.

vCare Features:

* Integrates eligibility, provider and claims information to improve workflow in UM, CM and DM

* Houses all of the necessary guidelines and requirements for UM, CM and DM

* Documents users' workflow within UM, CM and DM through an auditing function

vCare Benefits:

* One-stop shop for medical management

* Reduces unnecessary data entry

* Increases system connectivity

* Improves continuity within the coordination of care

* Meets National Committee for Quality Assurance (NCQA) requirements

In the final analysis, any population health and care management technology should be directed at improving health outcomes and lowering costs. These solutions, like Valence Health vCare© (see the sidebar, vCare's Approach to Case Management), also need to help make your PSHP's medical management processes operate more efficiently and effectively. Like any investment your PSHP makes, the return may take time, but will hopefully set your plan apart from its competitors, and help you to engender greater loyalty and support from your members and network providers.

Health Plan Internet Portals

The goal of portal technology is to enrich the user's experience and save your plan money by enabling self-service. With it, individuals do not have to make a phone call and wait on hold to get the answer to their questions; they can answer it themselves. By decreasing the customer service representatives' (CSRs) workload, your plan can free up time for these professionals to focus on more complex inquiries.

Health insurance portals further allow members, providers, brokers and employers to access and interact online with nearly real-time healthcare and insurance information. In making portal selection decisions, it is important for your PSHP to clearly classify its target stakeholders (as doing so will lead to better definition of the portal's features, functions, content and system integration requirements). For example, if your PSHP only offers Medicare Advantage and Medicaid products where the state auto-enrolls members into your plan, then you will not need a broker portal.

Since health plan stakeholders access portals for different reasons, know that if you want to encourage and increase portal use, these online interfaces should reflect this difference in stakeholder portal usage needs (for details surrounding different types of portal content and functionality, refer to Figure 12.4). Additionally, health plan portals need clearly defined governance structures, which are the sets of processes and procedures that will support your portals' ongoing operations and management.

Common Health Plan Web Portal Functionality

Source: Valence Health

Online portals are used by multiple different stakeholders to view specific content or complete a variety of tasks:

Stakeholder	Typical Content	Expected Tasks
Members	• Claims/Explanation of Benefits (EOB) • Account Balances/Accumulators • Demographics • Eligibility • Primary Care Physicians • Other Coverage • Pending/Open Requests • Invoices	• Edit Demographics • Add Dependents • Terminate or Extend Coverage • Change Primary Care Physician • Request ID Card/Print Temporary ID Card • Pay Premiums • Track Benefits Usage • Access Health and Wellness Tools • Research Cost of Care Data • Search for In-Network Hospitals and Providers • View Claims and Invoices • Submit Questions or Concerns • Schedule Appointments • Check Test Results
Employer	• Current Employee Roster • EOB • Plan Trend Analysis • Invoices • Employees' Information (Demographics, Eligibility, Primary Care Physician) • Other Coverage and Pending/Open Requests	• Edit Demographics • Add Dependents • Terminate Coverage • Change Primary Care Physician • Request ID Card/Print Temporary ID Card • Submit Questions or Concerns
Provider	• Claims • EOB • Explanation of Payment • Account Balances/Accumulators • Primary Care Physician Assignments • Other Coverage • Pending/Open Requests • Compliance with Care Guidelines and Incentive Programs	• View Patient Roster • View Remittance Advice • Check Medical Necessity Screening Criteria • Create, Submit, Edit, Check or Inquire about Authorizations • Submit and/or Obtain Appeals and Panel Reports • Confirm Member Eligibility, Benefits Summary and Effective Dates • Submit and Check Status of Claims and Authorizations
Broker	• Commissions • Plan Trend Analysis • Group/Employers • Group Information • Information for Employees with their Groups and Members/Individuals • Group/Individual Assignment by Broker	• Edit Demographics • Add Dependents • Terminate Coverage • Change Primary Care Physician Assignment • Request ID Card/Print Temporary ID Card • Submit Questions or Concerns

Figure 12.4

Depending on your execution strategy (as described in Chapter 3, "Determining Your PSHP's Comprehensive Execution Strategy"), your PSHP will know if it is wise to either develop and implement custom-built portals or commercial off-the-self portal software. The different types of portal software available will vary in their level of configuration, presence of controls and related support staff to help with your portal's development, maintenance, enhancements and upgrades.

Your plan's portals also can be used as a tool to improve member engagement. Your staff can track usage rate by user ID to identify which areas of the portal are heavily trafficked and by whom. With that information, your management team can strategically execute system revisions and develop new outreach programs to prioritize system improvements and promote greater portal adoption among targeted users (see Figure 12.5).

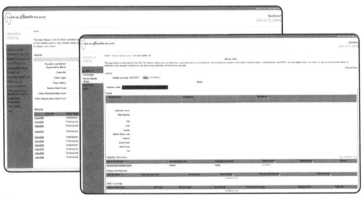

Examples of Provider and Member Portals Developed by Valence Health for Land of Lincoln Health

Source: Valence Health

Figure 12.5

While all portals can be powerful platforms to meet the growing desire for self-education and self-service, they do not replace personal interactions. Although portals may expedite a PSHP's internal functions, they can never replace them. Therefore, it is essential that members or providers always have a CSR that they can speak with.

Claim Processing Technology

In an insurer's claims payment process, everything runs through a system or technology platform. This system does the majority of work as long as it is robust enough and has the right protocols and management criteria built into it. All of the algorithms that are used for managing claims will use your PSHP's predetermined reimbursement or contract rules. The technology's ability to apply those rules is what makes a claim come out correctly or incorrectly.

Common Claim Rules Addressed by Health Insurance Claims Editing Engines

- Correct and clear coding relationships
- Frequency that a service can be performed in a set period of time
- Correct and incorrect codes and modifiers for a given service
- Types of services that can be bundled together for payment
- Diagnoses required to confirm services are medically necessary
- Errors, such as duplicate claims or age-specific claims for members who are outside the specified age range

Source: Valence Health
Figure 12.6

Typically in the health insurance industry, claims processing systems are built around a core system or platform that can be modified by easily adding modules. All of these interconnected parts feed off one another to adjudicate a claim according to your plan's predetermined rules. For example, one part of your claim processing system will be a claims editing engine that can use "if-then" types of logic to define which characteristics a claim must meet in order to get paid (for more information, see Figure 12.6 and the case study, *Following Claims Rules*).

Case Study:
Following Claim Rules – *Valence Health*

"Claims rules must be set up in the claim system to ensure that an account can be properly adjudicated. Certain types of service combinations may be permitted on one type of claim, but not allowed on others.

Valence Health recently worked with a Medicaid client when the state Medicaid agency required all plans to started offering a new targeted case management behavioral health benefit. The benefit allowed the same CPT-4 code to be billed multiple times on the same date of service. Since a normal claim configuration would deny the three codes following the first instance as duplicate services for the same date of service, Valence Health successfully wrote new rules in its claims engine to meet these unique billing requirements. We also limited that configuration to specific claim types and specific codes to make sure the same rule did not create duplicate payments for other types of services."

– Joe Cecil
Executive Director of Operations, Valence Health

Once your claims editing engine verifies that a claim was billed correctly, the claims processing system uses a payment system solution to accurately price the claim for reimbursement. This system calculates payment for in-network and out-of-network claims according to the appropriate state, federal or contract-specific payments you have negotiated with your plan's providers.

Finally, reimbursement will then be delivered to the correct bank accounts, and the system will generate and distribute electronic remittance advice to the impacted parties along with an explanation of benefits (EOB) statement that further describes the payment.

The beauty of these system components is that technology does most of the work for you by auto-adjudicating larger amounts of your plan's claims. In these systems, a clean claim that is free of mistakes can run through the system and be paid without any staff involvement. This streamlined approach is what many health plans aim for since it can help maximize payment accuracy, while minimizing inconsistent, costly and time-consuming manual review.

Simply know that added automation results in increased cost. Successful PSHPs typically conduct return on investment (ROI) analyses to make sure continued claims processing automation aligns with their plans' guiding principles and operational improvement priorities. Therefore, as your management team evaluates your PSHP's execution strategy (refer to Chapter 3, "Developing Your PSHP's Comprehensive Execution Strategy" for more information), you too will have to wrestle with all of your build, buy or partner/outsource decisions as it relates to your plan's claims processing needs at its very onset of operations and throughout its life cycle.

Call Center Technologies

Call centers rely heavily upon technology to fulfill their goal of providing excellent customer service and fulfilling the callers' needs effectively. While health plan call centers' technology needs are largely no different than the call center technology needs in other industries, there are four key technologies you will need to become familiar with (if you are not already), which are described in Figure 12.7.

Best practice recommends that these pieces of technology should be integrated and available on the same platform to facilitate the customer service representatives' quick, convenient access to all necessary resources. This also allows automated call distributor (ACD) Systems, Customer Relationship Management (CRM) Solution and Integrated Voice Response (IVR) Systems to work in conjunction, enabling effective call routing and intelligent access to your plan's member, provider and broker information databases. Ultimately, these technologies should help CSRs effectively fulfill customers' needs, enhance their experience and optimize call center key performance indicators.

Major Call Center Technologies

Source: UnitedHealthcare

Type	Possible Applications for Health Plans (To Reduce Call Handling Times and Help Improve Customer Satisfaction)
Automated Call Distributor (ACD) Systems	• Routes the call to the most appropriate CSR given numerous factors like language proficiencies and previous plan interactions • Supports multi-channel routing, which allows the consumer to interact on preferred communication platforms (e.g., phone, email, texts)
Computer Telephony Integration (CTI)	• Integrates CSRs' desktop applications with the ACD system so customer data in the CRM automatically appears on the CSRs' screens • Allows interactions to flow more smoothly and be more personalized
Customer Relationship Management (CRM) Solution	• Contains a wealth of information, e.g., demographics, previous call history, past email communications, and claims status and enrollment and benefits information that can be used by CSRs to help address many of your plan's customers' needs and concerns
Integrated Voice Response (IVR) Systems	• Enables the playing of prerecorded messages about the health plan while callers are on hold • Allows customers to use the keypad or the voice recognition feature to gather information and complete steps via self-service • Offers customers who prefer to communicate directly with a CSR, but cannot remain on hold, with a callback feature • Allows customers to leave voicemails that can be automatically converted into support tickets, which are added to the CSRs' work queue • Measures customer satisfaction metrics through surveys

Figure 12.7

Some health plans also choose to invest in workforce optimization (WFO) or workforce management (WFM) software. This technology helps optimize performance metrics by recording CSR-customer interactions for quality purposes and using call data to develop more effective work schedules. By capturing call center interactions, managers can identify barriers to customer satisfaction and areas for staff to improve or be retrained. Some systems even allow managers to use customizable, dynamic call scripts that guide the CSRs' actions using real-time suggestions. This capability also facilitates staff collaboration when resolving challenging customer interactions or transferring calls to another staff member. By capturing call data, WFO and WFM software also can help predict trends in call volumes and schedule CSRs accordingly.

Whatever call center technologies and features your health plan selects, know that you will still need to offer your customers the opportunity to speak directly with a live CSR (see sidebar). Identifying the appropriately balance between these two customer service elements can create differentiation from your competitors, improve your customer satisfaction scores and build customer loyalty.

Business Intelligence and Analytics Tools

To evaluate key retrospective and prospective business metrics, health plans generally use business intelligence (BI) tools (see Figure 12.8 for an example). These tools collect, organize and analyze integrated data sets to let your executive team know how well your health plan's products are performing. Depending upon the BI tools you select, your plan will be able to run a host of both standard and customized reports.

For more casual BI users, preexisting report templates with a standard list of fields allow individuals to query, filter and drill down into data. More advanced users can capitalize on more flexible, ad-hoc reporting capabilities that allow them to modify the reports' parameters and filters as needed (see Figure 12.9)

Inpatient Snapshot

Source: Valence Health vQuest© PSHP Standard Reporting Package

Inpatient Metrics

	Current Year					
	Admits/1,000	ALOS	Days/1,000	Paid/Day	Paid/Admit	PMPM
Acute Medical	43	4.3	185	$1,227	$5,325	$18.92
Maternity	50	2.3	112	$991	$2,243	$9.27
Acute Surgical	7	4.7	32	$4,560	$21,376	$12.10
Rehab/SNF	0		0			$0.00
MH/SA	5	7.1	33	$421	$3,002	$1.17
Total Inpatient	**104**	**3.5**	**362**	**$1,373**	**$4,798**	**$41.46**

Figure 12.8

Inpatient Snapshot *(cont.)*

Inpatient Metrics

	Year-Over-Year Trend					
	Admits/1,000	ALOS	Days/1,000	Paid/Day	Paid/Admit	PMPM
Acute Medical	(7%)	(4%)	(11%)	(15%)	(18%)	(24%)
Maternity	(16%)	(3%)	(18%)	(4%)	(7%)	(22%)
Acute Surgical	47%	5%	54%	(4%)	1%	48%
Rehab/SNF	(100%)		(100%)			(100%)
MH/SA	(21%)	(8%)	(28%)	(6%)	(14%)	(32%)
Total Inpatient	(10%)	(2%)	(12%)	**1%**	(1%)	(11%)

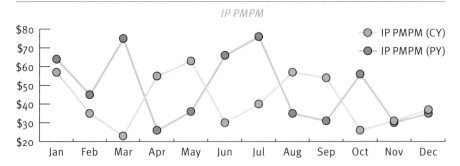

IP PMPM

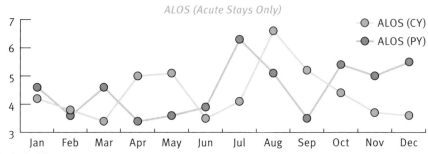

ALOS (Acute Stays Only)

Product = All
Current Year (CY): January 2012 to December 2012
Prior Year (PY): January 2011 to December 2011
SNF = Skilled Nursing Facility
MH = Mental Health
SA = Substance Abuse
ALOS = Average Length of Stay
PMPM = Per-Member-Per-Month
IP = Inpatient

Figure 12.8

The diverse functionalities that are present in many tools allow health plans to monitor compliance with evidence-based guidelines, and direct improvement initiatives by using current and past data to evaluate programs and tactics. Your BI tools ultimately can be used for multiple purposes including quality reporting, physician incentive design work, population health management, financial analysis and financial reporting.

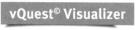

Source: Valence Health

Member contribution to total per-member-per-month (PMPM) spend grouped by the number of chronic conditions members have.

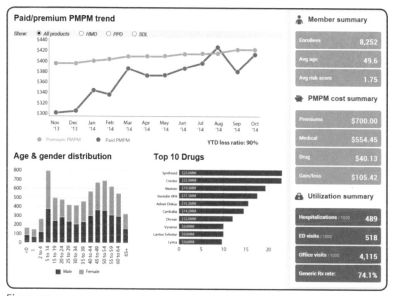

Figure 12.9

For example, management reports can function as executive-level dashboards that examine key plan operational health metrics, including per-member-per-month (PMPM) medical expense summaries, PMPM expenses by primary care provider specialty and monthly claims summary statistics. These reports can help staff identify outliers and identify the best approach for process improvements.

As a provider-sponsored health plan, you will need to better understand how to tweak aspects of the plan and program design to achieve better clinical and financial outcomes. As Valence Health developed vQuest©, its own BI solution, we have taken great care to make sure we can help our clients always be in a position where they can:

- Analyze medical costs and trends
- Stratify and prioritize patients

- Track medical loss ratio performance

- Observe readmission rates and average length of stay

- Compare cost over time versus benchmarks

- Perform predictive modeling for defined populations

- Track medical expenses across categories

- Profile physician performance on cost, utilization and quality

- Identify cost drivers and key performance indicators

- Benchmark productivity at the provider, practice or entity level

- Apply specialty profiles to patient care and network protocols to encourage compliance

- Make the case for care model changes

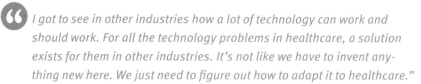

I got to see in other industries how a lot of technology can work and should work. For all the technology problems in healthcare, a solution exists for them in other industries. It's not like we have to invent anything new here. We just need to figure out how to adapt it to healthcare."

– Dan Blake
Chief Technology Officer, Valence Health

In its totality, the technology that your PSHP adopts or accesses through its partners needs to be viewed as a core capability. You will not be able to effectively compete with other plans or meet the ever increasing, technology-enabled demands of your customers unless you are keeping one eye focused on potential future technology supports that could help your PSHP fulfill its mission and adhere to its guiding principles.

Valence Health also has learned that healthcare technology advances and adaptations can move more quickly and efficiently by learning from other industries. ⊘

Tracking Key Health Plan Technology Metrics

Performing regular data analysis can help your PSHP maximize its return on investment and identify both early warning signs of trouble and indicators of success. By tracking key inputs and outputs, you can continually enhance your health plan so it retains members, remains financially stable and earns high patient satisfaction scores. Below are key health plan technology metrics that should be measured continuously:

- Patient outcomes
- Hospital readmission rates
- Healthcare expenses
- Providers' quality metrics
- Population health metrics
- Member risk scores
- Case management completion and abandonment rates
- Providers' administrative requirements for completing or fulfilling required health plan requirements
- Plan rates

- Plan profitability metrics
- Organization's financial stability metrics
- Cost and flexibility of technological upgrades
- Technology costs and expected ROI
- Patient and provider satisfaction rates
- Quality of customer service
- Claims processing accuracy
- Portal usage statistics by stakeholder
- Customer loyalty metrics
- Member engagement statistics

Industry Terminology Related to Technology

Automated Call Distributor (ACD)   A phone system that performs four basic functions: answers incoming calls, gets information and instructions from database, determines the best way to handle the call and sends the call to the proper agent, as soon as one is available.

Source: Genesys

Business Intelligence (BI)   A collection of computer-based techniques used in extracting, identifying and analyzing business data. BI technologies provide current and predictive views of business operations. Common functions of BI technologies are reporting, online analytical processing, data mining and more. Its aim is to support better business decision-making and, as a result, a BI system also can be known as a decision support system.

Source: Healthcare IT Index

Care Plan   A document that identifies healthcare orders for a patient and serves as a guide to care. It can either be written for an individual patient, be retrieved from a computer and individualized or be preprinted for a specific disease, condition or diagnosis and individualized to the specific patient. Standardized care plans are available for a number of patient conditions.

Source: "Miller-Keane Encyclopedia and Dictionary of Medicine, Nursing and Allied Health,"
Seventh Edition

Case Management   A collaborative process that helps consumers manage their comprehensive health needs through communication and available resources to promote quality, cost-effective outcomes. A health professional case manager assesses, plans, implements, coordinates, monitors and evaluates options for consumers, their families, caregivers and the healthcare team, including providers, to promote these outcomes.

Source: Utilization Review Accreditation Commission

Claim   A request for payment that you or your healthcare provider submits to your health insurer when you get items or services you think are covered.

Source: Healthcare.gov

Claim Adjudication   The determination of the insurer's payment or financial responsibility after the member's insurance benefits are applied to a medical claim.

Source: Medicaloffice.about.com

Customer Service Representative   Employee responsible for maintaining goodwill between a business organization and its customers by answering questions, solving problems and providing advice or assistance in utilizing the goods or services of the organization.

Source: AllBusiness.com

Denied Claim   The refusal of an insurance company or carrier to honor a request by an individual (or his or her provider) to pay for healthcare services obtained from a healthcare professional.

Source: Healthinsurance.org

Disease Management   Refers to the processes and people concerned with improving or maintaining health in large populations. It is concerned with common chronic illnesses and the reduction of future complications associated with those diseases.

Source: Utilization Review Accreditation Commission

Electronic Remittance Advice   A transaction that provides an electronic version of an explanation of payment and contains detailed information regarding a provider's adjudicated claim.

Source: American Medical Association

Explanation of Benefits (EOB)   A statement sent by a health insurance company to covered individuals explaining what medical treatments and/or services were paid for on their behalf.

Source: Valence Health

Health Risk Assessment (HRA)   A collection of health-related data that a provider can use to evaluate the health status and the health risk of an individual. The HRA will identify health behaviors and risk factors known only to the patient (e.g., physical activity and nutritional habits) for which the medical provider can provide tailored feedback in an approach to reduce the risk factors as well as the potential inevitability of the diseases to which they are related.

Source: CMS.gov

Hospital Admissions, Discharge and Transfer (ADT) System   A software system used by healthcare facilities in the U.S. to track patients from the point of arrival at a hospital until departure by transfer, discharge or death.

Source: Medical-dictionary.thefreedictionary.com

Interactive Voice Response (IVR)   A system that uses responses from a touch-tone telephone to gather and store data. It uses a human voice to read back. When set up with voice recognition software, data can be gathered through voice instead of touch tone.

Source: Genesys

Interoperability   The ability of different information technology systems and software applications to communicate, exchange data and use the information that has been exchanged.

Source: Healthcare Information Management Systems Society

Prior Authorization   Approval from a health plan that may be required before a member gets a service or fills a prescription in order for the service or prescription to be covered by their plan.

Source: HealthCare.gov

Telehealth   The use of electronic information and telecommunications technologies to support long-distance clinical healthcare, patient and professional health-related education, and public health and health administration. Technologies include videoconferencing, the Internet, store-and-forward imaging, streaming media and terrestrial and wireless communications.

Source: U.S. Department of Health and Human Services

Utilization Management   The evaluation of the medical necessity, appropriateness and efficiency of the use of healthcare services, procedures and facilities under the provisions of the applicable health benefits plan, sometimes called "utilization review."

Source: Utilization Review Accreditation Commission

Workforce Management (WFM)   An integrated set of processes that an institution uses to optimize the productivity of its employees on the individual, departmental and entity-wide levels. Also synonymous with Workforce Optimization Software (WFO).

Source: TechTarget

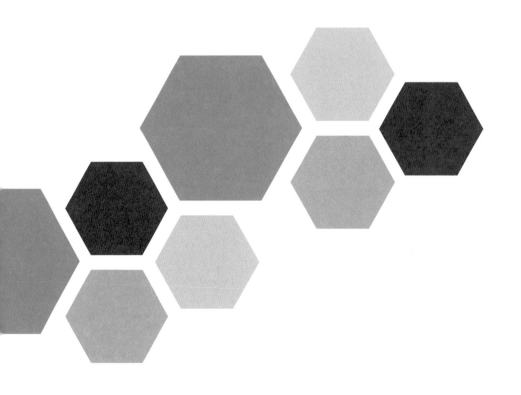

Glossary
Industry Terminology

Accreditation   Process in which a state or other standard-setting regulatory organization determines whether an entity seeking to provide services subject to that organization's authority meets acceptable standards for such purposes. For example, commercial insurers domiciled in a state that passes all the National Association of Insurance Commissioners (NAIC) model acts and otherwise passes muster will be acceptable security in other states.

Source: National Association of Insurance Commissioners

Actuarial Risk   A statistical method of estimating the risk of a particular event's occurrence (e.g., the risk of inpatient hospital admission). Actuarial methods are touted as more accurate than clinical judgment alone.

Source: Valence Health

Actuarial Value   The percentage of total average costs for covered benefits that a plan will cover. For example, if a plan has an actuarial value of 70%, on average, you would be responsible for 30% of the costs of all covered benefits. However, you could be responsible for a higher or lower percentage of the total costs of covered services for the year, depending on your actual healthcare needs and the terms of your insurance policy.

Source: HealthCare.gov

Administrative Fees   Payment for those business expenses that health plans incur when managing the non-clinical aspects of your health plan, e.g., printing membership cards, personnel and systems related to provider and member customer service portals, or overhead expenses.

Source: Valence Health

Appeal   A request for your health insurer or plan to review a decision or a grievance again.

Source: HealthCare.gov

Asset Risk   Risk related to market changes or poor investment performance of a financial asset (e.g., shares, options, futures or currency).

Source: RiskyThinking.com

Authorized Control Level Risk-Based Capital   Theoretical amount of capital plus surplus an insurance company should maintain.

Source: National Association of Insurance Commissioners

Automated Call Distributor (ACD)   A phone system that performs four basic functions: answers incoming calls, gets information and instructions from database, determines the best way to handle the call and sends the call to the proper agent, as soon as one is available.

Source: Genesys

Benefit   A service covered by a member's health insurance.

Source: The California Department of Managed Healthcare

Brokers   An insurance broker sells, solicits or negotiates insurance for compensation.

Source: Valence Health

Business Intelligence (BI)   A collection of computer-based techniques used in extracting, identifying and analyzing business data. BI technologies provide current and predictive views of business operations. Common functions of BI technologies are reporting, online analytical processing, data mining and more. Its aim is to support better business decision-making and, as a result, a BI system also can be known as a decision support system.

Source: Healthcare IT Index

Business Risk   The probability of loss inherent in an organization's operations and environment (such as competition and adverse economic conditions) that may impair its ability to provide returns on investment. Business risk plus the financial risk arising from use of debt (borrowed capital and/or trade credit) equal total corporate risk.

Source: BusinessDictionary.com

Capital   Wealth in the form of money or assets, taken as a sign of the financial strength of an individual, organization or nation, and assumed to be available for development or investment.

Source: BusinessDictionary.com

Capitation   A specified amount of money paid to a health plan or doctor. This is used to cover the cost of a health plan member's healthcare services for a certain length of time.

Source: CMS.gov

Care Coordination   The deliberate organization of patient care activities between two or more participants (including the patient) involved in a patient's care to facilitate the appropriate delivery of healthcare services. Organizing care involves the marshalling of personnel and other resources needed to carry out all required patient care activities, and is often managed by the exchange of information among participants responsible for different aspects of care.

Source: Agency for Healthcare Research and Quality

Care Plan A document that identifies healthcare orders for a patient and serves as a guide to care. It can either be written for an individual patient, be retrieved from a computer and individualized or be preprinted for a specific disease, condition or diagnosis and individualized to the specific patient. Standardized care plans are available for a number of patient conditions.

Source: "Miller-Keane Encyclopedia and Dictionary of Medicine, Nursing and Allied Health," Seventh Edition

Carriers A commercial enterprise licensed in a state to sell insurance.

Source: Valence Health

Carve-Outs Health insurance carve-outs concern a method to separate specific services from general healthcare contracts. A different contract and payment arrangement covers the designated "carved-out" services. Carve-outs also include services or benefits provided to a smaller segment of an employee population, or used to offer additional benefits under a different insurance carrier.

Source: eHow.com

Case Management A collaborative process that helps consumers manage their comprehensive health needs through communication and available resources to promote quality, cost-effective outcomes. A health professional case manager assesses, plans, implements, coordinates, monitors and evaluates options for consumers, their families, caregivers and the healthcare team, including providers, to promote these outcomes.

Source: Utilization Review Accreditation Commission

Claim A request for payment that you or your healthcare provider submits to your health insurer when you get items or services you think are covered.

Source: Healthcare.gov

Claim Adjudication The determination of the insurer's payment or financial responsibility after the member's insurance benefits are applied to a medical claim.

Source: Medicaloffice.about.com

Coinsurance The patient's share of the costs for a covered healthcare service, calculated as a percent (for example, 20%) of the allowed amount for the service. The member pays coinsurance plus any deductibles they may owe. For example, if the health insurance or plan's allowed amount for an office visit is $100 and the patient met the deductible, his coinsurance payment of 20% would be $20. Your health insurance plan pays the rest of the allowed amount.

Source: HealthCare.gov

Comorbidity The simultaneous presence of two chronic diseases or conditions in a patient.

Source: Merriam-Webster

Complication Allowance   When using bundled payments for reimbursement, some contracts include an ability to distinguish routine costs of care from costs associated with complications. These complications can become part of a warranty allowance that is built into each bundled payment and thus creates a margin opportunity for the participating providers.

Source: Health Care Incentives Improvement Institute

Consumer Assessment of Healthcare Providers and Systems (CAHPS) Surveys that ask consumers and patients to report on and evaluate their experiences with healthcare. These surveys focus on aspects of quality that consumers are best qualified to assess, such as the communication skills of providers and ease of access to healthcare services.

Source: Agency for Healthcare Research and Quality

Continuity of Care   Continuity of care is concerned with quality of care over time. It is the process by which the patient and his/her physician-led care team are cooperatively involved in ongoing healthcare management toward the shared goal of high quality, cost-effective medical care.

Source: American Academy of Family Physicians

Continuum of Care   A concept involving a system that guides and tracks patients over time through a comprehensive array of health services spanning all levels and intensity of care. The continuum of care covers the delivery of healthcare over a period of time, and may refer to care provided from birth to end of life. Healthcare services are provided for all levels and stages of care.

Source: Healthcare Information Management Systems Society

Coordination of Benefits (COB)   A way to figure out who pays first when two or more health insurance plans are responsible for paying the same medical claim.

Source: HealthCare.gov

Copay   A fixed amount (for example, $15) the member pays for a covered healthcare service, usually when the service is delivered. The amount also can vary by the type of covered healthcare service. Outpatient office visits may have a $25 copay, while emergency room visits could have a $150 copay.

Source: HealthCare.gov

Cost-Sharing   The share of costs covered by the member's insurance that the member pays out of his/her own pocket. This term generally includes deductibles, coinsurance and copayments or similar charges, but it does not include premiums, balance billing amounts for non-network providers or the cost of non-covered services. Cost-sharing in Medicaid and the Children's Health Insurance Program also includes premiums.

Source: HealthCare.gov

Credit Risk   Probability of loss from a debtor's default. In banking, credit risk is a major factor in determination of interest rate on a loan; the longer the term of the loan, usually the higher the interest rate.

Source: BusinessDictionary.com

Customer Service Representative   Employee responsible for maintaining goodwill between a business organization and its customers by answering questions, solving problems and providing advice or assistance in utilizing the goods or services of the organization.

Source: AllBusiness.com

Deductible   The amount patients owe for healthcare services before their health insurance or plan begins to pay. For example, if your deductible is $1,000, your plan will not cover anything until you have paid that full amount. The deductible, however, may not apply to all services. For example, an annual physical will be paid for regardless if you have spent $1,000 on other covered services.

Source: HealthCare.gov

Denied Claim   The refusal of an insurance company or carrier to honor a request by an individual (or his or her provider) to pay for healthcare services obtained from a healthcare professional.

Source: Healthinsurance.org

Disease Management   Refers to the processes and people concerned with improving or maintaining health in large populations. It is concerned with common chronic illnesses and the reduction of future complications associated with those diseases.

Source: Utilization Review Accreditation Commission

Electronic Medical Record   A real-time patient health record with access to evidence-based decision support tools that can be used to aid clinicians in decision making. The EMR can automate and streamline a clinician's workflow, ensuring that all clinical information is communicated. It can also prevent delays in response that result in gaps in care. The EMR can also support the collection of data for uses other than clinical care, such as billing, quality management, outcome reporting and public health disease surveillance and reporting. Synonymous with Electronic Health Record or EHR.

Source: Office of the National Coordinator for Health IT

Electronic Remittance Advice   A transaction that provides an electronic version of an explanation of payment and contains detailed information regarding a provider's adjudicated claim.

Source: American Medical Association

Eligibility Entitlement of an individual to receive services based on that individual's enrollment in a healthcare plan.

Source: Mosby's Medical Dictionary, 8th edition

Equity Net worth of a person or company computed by subtracting total liabilities from the total assets.

Source: BusinessDictionary.com

Evidence-Based Practices Applying the best available research results (evidence) when making decisions about healthcare. Healthcare professionals who perform evidence-based practice use research evidence along with clinical expertise and patient preferences.

Source: Effectivehealthcare.AHRQ.gov

Explanation of Benefits (EOB) A statement sent by a health insurance company to covered individuals explaining what medical treatments and/or services were paid for on their behalf.

Source: Valence Health

Gated and Ungated Care In the insurance industry, "gated" generically describes a plan that requires a referral from a primary care physician before a patient can visit a specialist. The doctor, his/her staff and the insurance company are positioned as gatekeepers to eliminate unnecessary testing and procedures. The cost of gated health insurance plans is less than non-gated plans, ones that allow customers to freely seek services from a specialist. Non-gated health insurance policies are more flexible, and as such usually demand higher premiums.

Source: eHow.com

Grievance A grievance is any complaint or dispute (other than an organization determination) expressing dissatisfaction with any aspect of the operations, activities or behavior of a health plan or its providers, regardless of whether remedial action is requested. The enrollee must file the grievance either orally or in writing no later than 60 days after the triggering event or incident precipitating the grievance.

Source: CMS.gov

Healthcare Effectiveness Data and Information Set (HEDIS) A tool used by more than 90% of America's health plans to measure performance on important dimensions of care and service. Altogether, HEDIS consists of 81 measures across five domains of care. Because so many plans collect HEDIS data, and because the measures are so specifically defined, HEDIS makes it possible to compare the performance of health plans on an "apples-to-apples" basis.

Source: National Committee for Quality Assurance

Health Information Exchange (HIE) The electronic movement of health-related information among organizations according to nationally recognized standards. The goal of health information exchange is to facilitate access to and retrieval of clinical data to provide safer, timelier, efficient, effective, equitable and patient-centered care.

Source: U.S. Department of Health and Human Services

Health Maintenance Organization (HMO) A type of health insurance plan that usually limits coverage to care from doctors who work for or contract with the HMO. It generally will not cover out-of-network care except in an emergency. An HMO may require you to live or work in its service area to be eligible for coverage. HMOs often provide integrated care and focus on prevention and wellness.

Source: HealthCare.gov

Health Risk Assessment (HRA) A collection of health-related data that a provider can use to evaluate the health status and the health risk of an individual. The HRA will identify health behaviors and risk factors known only to the patient (e.g., physical activity and nutritional habits) for which the medical provider can provide tailored feedback in an approach to reduce the risk factors as well as the potential inevitability of the diseases to which they are related.

Source: CMS.gov

Health Savings Account (HSA) A medical savings account available to taxpayers who are typically enrolled in a high-deductible health plan. The funds contributed to the account are not subject to federal income tax at the time of deposit. Funds must be used to pay for qualified medical expenses. Funds roll over year to year if they are not spent.

Source: HealthCare.gov

High-Dollar Claims Expensive health services such as organ transplants or long-term cancer treatments.

Source: HHC Insurance Holdings, Inc.

Hospital Admissions, Discharge and Transfer (ADT) System A software system used by healthcare facilities in the U.S. to track patients from the point of arrival at a hospital until departure by transfer, discharge or death.

Source: Medical-dictionary.thefreedictionary.com

Indemnity Plan A type of health plan under which a covered person must pay 100% of all covered charges up to the plan's annual deductible. Once the deductible is met, a percentage of the covered charges must be paid by the covered person, up to the plan's out-of-pocket maximum. Indemnity plans do not usually offer in- or out-of-network benefit restrictions, but out-of-pocket costs are usually less when services are received by in-network healthcare professionals.

Source: Cigna.com/glossary

Independent Practice Association (IPA) A legal entity organized and directed by physicians in private practice to negotiate contracts with insurance companies on their behalf. Participating physicians are usually paid on a capitated or modified fee-for-service basis and may also continue to care for patients not covered by the insurers with whom the IPA contracts. Perhaps the most significant function of an IPA is to exert influence on behalf of its members to counterbalance the leverage of healthcare insurers. Synonymous with Independent Physicians Association.

Source: RiverCity Medical Group

Interactive Voice Response (IVR)   A system that uses responses from a touch-tone telephone to gather and store data. It uses a human voice to read back. When set up with voice recognition software, data can be gathered through voice instead of touch tone.

Source: Genesys

Interoperability   The ability of different information technology systems and software applications to communicate, exchange data and use the information that has been exchanged.

Source: Healthcare Information Management Systems Society

License   Certification of appropriate authority issued by a regulatory body to allow an entity to operate as an insurer or an insurance agent after certain standards have been met.

Source: International Risk Management Institute

Medicaid A state-administered health insurance program for low-income families and children, pregnant women, the elderly, people with disabilities and in some states, other adults. The federal government provides a portion of the funding for Medicaid and sets guidelines for the program.

Source: HealthCare.gov

Medicaid Expansion   The Affordable Care Act provides states with additional federal funding to expand their Medicaid programs to cover adults under 65 with income up to 133% of the federal poverty level. Children (18 and under) are eligible up to that income level or higher in all states. This means that in states that have expanded Medicaid, free or low-cost health coverage is available to people with incomes below a certain level regardless of disability, family status, financial resources and other factors that are usually taken into account in Medicaid eligibility decisions.

Source: Healthcare.gov

Medical Management   An umbrella term that includes utilization management, case management and disease management functions. Medical management strategies and programs are designed to improve population health by guiding consumer and/or provider behavior toward the healthiest options. Also synonymous with Medical Cost Management.

Source: Valence Health

Medical Diagnosis-Related Group   Under Medicare's inpatient prospective payment system, each case is categorized into a diagnosis-related group (DRG), which has a payment weight assigned to it based on the average resources used to treat Medicare patients in that group.

Source: CMS.gov

Medicare   A federal health insurance program for people who are age 65 or older and certain younger people with disabilities. It also covers people with End-Stage Renal Disease (permanent kidney failure requiring dialysis or a transplant, sometimes called ESRD).

Source: HealthCare.gov

Medicare Advantage   A type of Medicare health plan offered by a private company that contracts with Medicare to provide you with all your Part A and Part B benefits. Medicare Advantage plans include HMOs, PPOs, private FFS plans, Special Needs Plans and Medicare Medical Savings Account Plans. Most Medicare Advantage plans offer prescription drug coverage.

Source: HealthCare.gov

Medicare Advantage Star Rating System   Medicare uses a Star Rating System to measure how well Medicare Advantage and prescription drug (Part D) plans perform. Medicare scores how well plans did in several categories, including quality of care and customer service. The overall star rating score provides a way to compare performance among several plans.

Source: MedicareInteractive.org

Narrow Network Health Plan   Limits providers to a select group to make costs more affordable to members.

Source: NYTimes.com

National Association of Insurance Commissioners (NAIC)   The U.S. standard-setting and regulatory support organization created and governed by the chief insurance regulators from the 50 states, the District of Columbia and five U.S. territories. Through the NAIC, state insurance regulators establish standards and best practices, conduct peer review and coordinate their regulatory oversight.

Source: NAIC

National Committee for Quality Assurance (NCQA)   A nonprofit organization, the NCQA seal is a widely recognized symbol of quality. Organizations incorporating the seal into advertising and marketing materials must first pass a rigorous, comprehensive review and must annually report on their performance.

Source: NCQA.org

Open Enrollment   A period of time, usually but not always occurring once per year, when employees of companies and organizations may make changes to their elected fringe benefit options, such as health insurance. The term also applies to the annual period during which individuals may buy individual health insurance plans through the online, state-based health insurance exchanges established by the Patient Protection and Affordable Care Act.

Source: Wikipedia.org

Per-Member-Per-Month (PMPM)   Refers to the ratio of a service or cost divided by the number of members in a group. For example, if 10,000 members of an HMO had $20,000 in spending for cardiovascular surgery, the cost per member would be $2 per month.

Source: American Academy of Family Physicians

Point of Service (POS)   A type of plan in which you pay less if you use doctors, hospitals and other healthcare providers that belong to the plan's network. POS plans also require you to get a referral from your primary care doctor in order to see a specialist.

Source: HealthCare.gov

Practice Management Systems   A tool or type of software to help manage day-to-day operations in physicians' offices. These systems are often used for financial and administrative functions, and can also be linked with a patient's health or dental record. Practice management software can help track billing and demographic data, along with appointment scheduling.

Source: U.S. Department of Health and Human Services

Preferred Provider Organization (PPO)   A type of health plan that contracts with medical providers, such as hospitals and doctors, to create a network of participating providers. You pay less if you use providers that belong to the plan's network. You can use doctors, hospitals and providers outside of the network for an additional cost.

Source: HealthCare.gov

Premium   The amount that must be paid by the insured for his/her health insurance or plan. The member or his/her employers usually pay the premium monthly, quarterly or yearly.

Source: HealthCare.gov

Primary Coverage   If a person is covered under more than one health insurance plan, primary coverage is the coverage provided by the health insurance plan that pays on claims first.

Source: eHealth

Prior Authorization   Approval from a health plan that may be required before members get a service or fills a prescription in order for the service or prescription to be covered by their plan.

Source: HealthCare.gov

Quaternary Care   Very specialized and highly unusual care that is not offered in every hospital or medical setting, e.g., experimental medicine and procedures or highly uncommon, specialized surgeries.

Source: Patients.About.com

Reserves   The money a company or individual keeps on-hand to meet its short-term and emergency funding needs.

Source: Investopedia.com

Return on Investment (ROI)   A performance measure used to evaluate the efficiency of an investment or to compare the efficiency of a number of different investments.

Source: Investopedia.com

Risk-Based Capital (RBC)   In health insurance, RBC rules establish the minimum required liquid assets or cash reserves that health plans must have on-hand. Risk-based capital requirements exist to protect the firms, their investors and customers and the economy as a whole. Placement of risk-based capital requirements ensure that each financial institution has enough capital to sustain operating losses, while maintaining a safe and efficient market.

Source: Investopedia.com/terms

Risk Score   In a typical health risk assessment, each individual is scored based on an algorithm that incorporates information on the individual's age, any illnesses during the previous year and other factors. Patients' responses to health questions generate a numerical value, which is combined to produce a risk score so that a weighted average value can be determined and used to compare the relative risk of one population to another.

Source: Actuary.com

Risk Stratification   A systematic process for identifying and predicting patient risk levels relating to healthcare needs, services and coordination. It involves use of algorithms and registries, payor data, physician/provider judgment/input and patient self-assessments and experiences.

Source: New Jersey Academy of Family Physicians

Secondary Coverage   When a person is covered under more than one health insurance plan, this term describes the health insurance plan that provides payment on claims after the primary coverage.

Source: eHealth

Stop-Loss Premium   The dollar amount of claims filed for eligible expenses at which point you have paid 100% of your out-of-pocket and the insurance begins to pay at 100%. Stop-loss is reached when an insured individual has paid the deductible and reached the out-of-pocket maximum amount of coinsurance.

Source: Healthinsurance.org

Telehealth   The use of electronic information and telecommunications technologies to support long-distance clinical healthcare, patient and professional health-related education, and public health and health administration. Technologies include videoconferencing, the Internet, store-and-forward imaging, streaming media and terrestrial and wireless communications.

Source: U.S. Department of Health and Human Services

Third-Party Administrator (TPA)   A person or organization that processes claims and performs other administrative services in accordance with a service contract, usually in the field of employee benefits. More specifically, a TPA is neither the insurer (provider) nor the insured (employees or plan participants), but handles the administration of the plan including processing, adjudication, and negotiation of claims, recordkeeping and maintenance of the plan.

Source: MyCafeteriaPlan.com

Underwriting Risk   The probability that an actual return on an investment will be lower than the expected return.

Source: BusinessDictionary.com

Uniform Certificate of Authority Application (UCAA)   A process designed to allow insurers to file copies of the same application for admission in numerous states. Each state that accepts the UCAA is designated as a uniform state. While each uniform state still performs its own independent review of each application, the need to file different applications, in different formats, has been eliminated for all states that accept the uniform application.

Source: National Association of Insurance Commissioners

Utilization Management   The evaluation of the medical necessity, appropriateness and efficiency of the use of healthcare services, procedures and facilities under the provisions of the applicable health benefits plan, sometimes called "utilization review."

Source: Utilization Review Accreditation Commission

Utilization Review Accreditation Commission (URAC)   An independent, non-profit organization, URAC is a well-known leader in promoting healthcare quality through its accreditation, education and measurement programs.

Source: URAC.org

Utilization Review Agent (URA)   People working on behalf of a health insurance company who review a request for medical treatment and confirm a health plan provides coverage for medical services. This helps the company minimize costs and determine if the recommended treatment is appropriate.

Source: Health.HowStuffWorks.com

Value-Based Care   Linking provider payments to improved performance by healthcare providers. This form of payment holds healthcare providers accountable for both the cost and quality of care they provide. It attempts to reduce inappropriate care and to identify and reward the best-performing providers.

Source: HealthCare.gov

Workforce Management (WFM)   An integrated set of processes that an institution uses to optimize the productivity of its employees on the individual, departmental and entity-wide levels. Also synonymous with Workforce Optimization Software (WFO).

Source: TechTarget

Wrap Network   Wrap networks provide access to in-network providers, hospitals and ancillary services throughout the nation, providing a broad network for when your members are out of area and require medical care. Most PSHPs form a single contract with a national preferred provider organization (PPO) network to form a wrap network. Plan members can identify the wrap network from their ID card and hopefully access the closest in-network provider.

Source: Valence Health

About the Authors

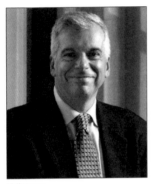

Phil Kamp
CEO and Co-Founder

Phil Kamp, Chief Executive Officer and Co-Founder, provides leadership and direction for Valence Health and leads the company's efforts in creating patient-focused, data-driven solutions that can be implemented across a healthcare organization.

Mr. Kamp has more than 30 years of managed care experience focusing on integration strategies for health systems. Since founding Valence Health, he has worked actively with physicians and healthcare executives in developing, implementing and managing clinically integrated and provider-sponsored risk-bearing organizations. These organizations have assumed varied levels of risk, from risk sharing to provider-sponsored health plans. In addition to his consulting experience, Mr. Kamp has served as the interim CEO and Chief Financial Officer of several provider-sponsored health plans.

Mr. Kamp's areas of expertise include strategic planning and business development, operational and financial management, development and financing of integrated delivery systems, compensation model design and implementation, and turnaround assistance for failing managed care plans.

Prior to co-founding Valence Health, Mr. Kamp was a Partner at Pricewaterhouse-Coopers, where he led the formation of numerous independent practice associations, physician hospital organizations and provider-sponsored health plans. He holds a Bachelor of Arts from Michigan State University and an MBA from Oakland University.

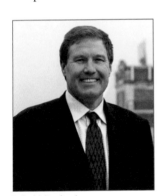

R. Todd Stockard
President and Co-Founder

R. Todd Stockard, President and Co-Founder of Valence Health, works with providers to develop and implement better patient care strategies, focusing on the development of clinical and financial-driven data models for managing provider-sponsored risk entities.

Mr. Stockard has more than 25 years of healthcare financial and data management experience. He actively works with providers and provider-sponsored health plans to develop, negotiate and operationalize value-based risk contracting agreements. He has used his information technology skills to develop and manage Valence Health's data management and analytic services for its clients.

Mr. Stockard's areas of expertise include: development of management reporting and physician-profiling systems for risk-bearing entities; creating financial feasibility studies for risk-assuming organizations; creating utilization and quality-based financial incentive models for provider full-risk managed care products; developing capitated pricing strategies; and analyzing claims databases to support both financial and utilization strategies for networks assuming risk.

Prior to co-founding Valence Health, Mr. Stockard was a senior manager in the managed care consulting group for PricewaterhouseCoopers. He holds a Bachelor of Arts in economics from Princeton University.

Phil Kamp and R. Todd Stockard co-founded Valence Health in 1997. In 2010, they were selected for induction into the 2010 Chicago Area Entrepreneurship Hall of Fame. In 2015, Valence Health was recognized by *Crain's Chicago Business* as being one of Chicago's Fast Fifty — one of the fastest-growing healthcare companies in Illinois. ⬡